The Definitive Guide to Thriving After Cancer

THE DEFINITIVE GUIDE TO
Thriving
After Cancer

A Five-Step Integrative Plan to
Reduce the Risk of Recurrence
and Build Lifelong Health

Lise N. Alschuler, ND, FABNO,
AND Karolyn A. Gazella

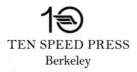

TEN SPEED PRESS
Berkeley

Published in the United States by Ten Speed Press, an imprint of the
Crown Publishing Group, a division of Random House LLC, a
Penguin Random House Company, New York.
www.crownpublishing.com
www.tenspeed.com

Ten Speed Press and the Ten Speed Press colophon are registered trademarks
of Random House LLC.

A previous edition of this work was published in the United States as
Five to Thrive: Your Cutting-edge Cancer Prevention Plan by Active Interest Media, Inc.,
El Segundo, California, in 2011.

Library of Congress Cataloging-in-Publication Data
Alschuler, Lise.
  [Five to thrive]
  The definitive guide to thriving after cancer : a five-step integrative plan to reduce
the risk of recurrence and build lifelong health / Lise N. Alschuler, ND, FABNO
and Karolyn A. Gazella. — Revised edition.
      pages cm
  Revision of: Five to thrive. — El Segundo, California : Active Interest, 2011.
(eBook) 1. Cancer—Diet therapy. 2. Cancer—Prevention. I. Gazella, Karolyn A.
II. Title.
  RC271.D52A43 2013
  616.99'40654—dc23
                                        2013014557

Trade Paperback ISBN: 978-1-60774-564-8
eBook ISBN: 978-1-60774-565-5

Printed in the United States of America

Design by Chloe Rawlins

10 9 8 7 6 5 4 3

Revised Edition

Contents

*When we think of the many Thrivers we have met along our journey,
our hearts expand. We are both humbled and exhilarated by their influence
on our work. To all of the Thrivers whose paths we have crossed, thank you;
and to all of the Thrivers we have not yet met, we can't wait to meet you!*

Preface

We have an intensely deep and personal connection to this illness. We are both cancer survivors and we have each lost a parent to cancer. In addition, we have a combined total of more than forty years in the natural health industry, focusing on patient education and patient care, with much of that time devoted to the investigation, practice, and advocacy of integrative cancer care. We have written this book specifically for people like us—people who want to proactively reduce their risk of a cancer recurrence. In talking with other survivors, we have found that people want straight answers and clear direction. People who have witnessed family members and friends go through this illness are motivated to avoid cancer and are seeking specific prevention strategies. This book answers that incredible need. The Five to Thrive Plan will not only reduce your risk of cancer, but it will also provide a blueprint for living a vibrantly healthy life.

The goal of this book is to help you create a path toward a deep-seated wellness that stays with you to your very last breath. That may sound lofty, but we will settle for nothing less. Before we ever wrote one word of our first book, *The Definitive Guide to Cancer*, we created a guiding vision and mission. Since then, we have begun every presentation and book with these statements:

Our Vision. An integrative approach to cancer prevention and treatment can positively transform the health of those affected by this disease.

Our Mission. By educating people about lifestyle-based, integrative, and scientifically sound health promotion strategies, we create deeper and more widespread wellness.

Developing the Five to Thrive Plan was a natural extension of our life's work toward the fulfillment of our vision and mission.

The inspiration for this second edition featuring the Five to Thrive Plan came from the readers of the first edition. We heard many stories of readers who were inspired anew to lead healthier lives. They told us how they shared our book with their book clubs and set up self-help groups. Some readers used our book as a part of their wellness coaching. From their feedback, we saw the opportunity to make the Five to Thrive Plan even easier to follow. This second edition is a call to action that is even more clear and concise. We are deeply grateful for the feedback that we have received, and we are honored to offer this new updated and improved edition.

We developed the Five to Thrive Plan with these goals in mind:

- Simple
- Practical
- Sustainable
- Backed by science, and
- Effective

As cancer survivors, we created this plan for ourselves and our loved ones, but we have always wanted this plan to be *yours*. A plan that you can individualize, customize, and mold into your own personal version of thriving. At the end of each chapter, you will find a Thrive Thought as well as some simple next steps. Think of these as steppingstones, with each stone bringing you one step closer to exuberant and vital wellness.

The Five to Thrive Plan

A cancer diagnosis delivers a breathtaking blow to body, mind, and spirit. It also comes with a huge dose of distraction as you are hurled into the world of cancer treatment. But what happens when the last round of treatment is completed, the doctor visits are few and far between, and the tests have all been taken? What then? We hear that question a lot. With a pat on the back and a sincere "good luck," people with a past diagnosis of cancer often feel unarmed as they move into their new life as a *cancer survivor*. They sense they are ill equipped to reduce their risk of recurrence—and yet the thought of having cancer again looms large. The reality that they are at a higher risk of getting cancer again is daunting.

Cancer is not something we *want* to think about, but even if we try to shove it back to the dark recesses of the mind, it is still there, niggling. Periodically, our fear thunders into our awareness, sending us into swirling panic. This can happen when we experience a new body ache, a day of unusual tiredness, or a stubborn mental block. It can crop up if we know someone in treatment, or even when we celebrate the anniversary of our diagnosis or our own treatment. At times, it can seem that we are dancing on ice, doing our best to avoid falling through, but without a clear sense of where the ice is thin and where the ice will hold us.

But in an ironic twist of truth, this illness—and the fear it evokes—can teach us how to embrace life, to meet it head on, and to live with vitality. The experience of confronting cancer can teach us how to reduce the risk of it returning. It can be a bridge to deeper and greater health. It is the Trojan horse for the real message of thriving. This call for vital living inspired us to write *The Definitive Guide to Thriving After Cancer*. During our many public presentations across the country, we have met hundreds of people who share more than the bond of cancer—they share the inspiring drive to triumph over adversity and fight not only for themselves but also for the people they love. As survivors of cancer ourselves, we have learned a lot from these courageous people. We have also heard their pleas for trustworthy guidance.

This book is a culmination of wisdom gleaned from our own experiences (both personal and clinical), the accounts of others who have walked with cancer on various levels, and a careful distilling of the available research and scientific literature. But most of all, this book is a lesson in *thriving*, with a clear picture of what that looks like and how to get there. Thriving is the perfect antidote to fear—and the key ingredient to living an exuberant life.

Thriving Versus Surviving

The Greek philosopher Aristotle once wrote: "The ultimate value of life depends upon awareness and the power of contemplation rather than upon mere survival." The fact that you're reading this book to begin with suggests you just might agree with Aristotle. In fact, few of us are content to just get by, especially when it comes to our health. Yet when we are in the throes of illness, mere survival may be an admirable goal. For some who have battled cancer—or fought alongside a loved one with cancer—simply surviving the fight is success.

Survivors emerge on the other side buoyed by love yet battle-fatigued. We know what it's like to move into survival mode. We understand the feeling of taking things one day at a time and, in the heat of battle, appreciating the smallest of victories. We understand the terror this illness brings. However, in these moments of fear we have the opportunity to achieve a deep awareness of what it takes to effectively transition from *survivor* to *Thriver*. Facing our cancer fears can create an opportunity to dive deeply into life to discover its true treasures. Thrivers embrace an intense yearning for vibrant health and vital living. We applaud your initiative in taking a proactive approach to your health. This book provides a practical, easy-to-use template to help you achieve your highest health goals and to experience life as it is meant to be experienced—with exhilaration, meaning, and joy!

The Five to Thrive Concept

At the core, cancer prevention is the act of proactively reducing one's risk of developing the illness. But we take our philosophy one step further. To us, this journey is about rediscovering vitality no matter what we encounter. The Five to Thrive Plan will make sure you're the healthiest you can be if ever you do develop cancer. It may seem counterintuitive, maybe even radical, to describe a person with cancer as *healthy*, but the most effective risk reduction plan also prepares your body for the *potential* of battle. We need to create a foundation for success against cancer. The Five to Thrive Plan helps you look at cancer prevention differently. We show you—based on scientific evidence—that you have the power to change the course of cancer development, and in doing so, to transform your health. The scientific concept of epigenetics (the science of examining factors that influence the behavior of our genes) continues to confirm that we can change the way our genes behave. We can, quite literally, transform our internal landscape, and our plan shows you how to do that.

We begin by identifying the body's five key pathways that have the most influence on whether we are healthy or become sick. These pathways are:

1. The immune system

2. Inflammation

3. Hormonal balance

4. Insulin resistance

5. Digestion and detoxification

The Five to Thrive Plan helps you enhance the immune system, reduce inflammation, sustain hormonal balance, prevent and reduce insulin resistance, and optimize digestion and detoxification.

These five key pathways in the body can be positively influenced by focusing on five core strategies:

1. Enhance your **spirit**

2. Let's **move**

3. Enrich your **diet**

4. Utilize **dietary supplements**

5. Create **rejuvenation**

As you can see from the illustration on the opposite page, within each of the five core strategies, there are five critical action steps. These actions steps have been prioritized based on their influence on the body's five key pathways. If an action positively impacts the five pathways, it becomes a priority within the Five to Thrive Plan. The connection between actions and impact must be validated by the scientific research in order to make it part of the plan. When you focus on the five critical action steps within each of these core strategies, you are positively affecting the function and health of all five pathways. As a result, you will significantly reduce your risk of developing cancer and live a more vibrantly healthy and joyful life.

The Five to Thrive Plan

Positively influence your pathways with these core strategies and action steps.

SPIRIT
Joy
Hope
Laughter
Service
Love

REJUVENATION
Rhythm
Rest
Relax
Replenish
Remediate

MOVEMENT
Muscle strengthening
Aerobic activity
Stretching and flexibility
Proper timing
Optimal hydration

HEALTH

Your body's
five key pathways:

1. The Immune System
2. Inflammation
3. Hormonal Balance
4. Insulin Resistance
5. Digestion and
   Detoxification

AND WELLNESS

DIETARY SUPPLEMENTS
Omega-3 fatty acids
Probiotics
Polyphenols
Antioxidants
Vitamin D

DIET
Engage your senses
Add more color
Eat organic
Eat more whole foods
Spice it up

As you can see, the number five is important to our plan. There are:

- Five key pathways
- Five core strategies, and
- Five critical action steps

Successfully Changing Behaviors

It's been said that the only constant in life is change. That can sometimes be maddening, but it will work in your favor as you change how you live your life. The key to behavior change is to become attached to the outcome, develop a solid plan, and then be gentle with yourself on days that you fall short. Eventually, and often sooner than you might imagine, you will find that the changes are no longer changes but have seamlessly become part of how you live day to day. In the process, you will discover that you have created an entirely new way of living.

The human body adapts to input it receives. For example, if you normally eat a diet comprised of healthy, organic, unprocessed whole foods and then, on a whim, eat several pieces of pizza and a pint of ice cream one night, you will feel the ill effects soon after. However, if you eat pizza and ice cream regularly, your body adjusts and will give up sending you warning signals. It will adapt to that diet. Fortunately, the body adapts just as surely to healthy changes. If you begin walking for thirty minutes four times a week, you will soon notice that you can increase to five times a week and even go a little longer or faster with ease. When walking becomes part of what's normal to your body, it "tells" you when you miss a day. Regular walkers often report feeling tired or lethargic or experiencing headaches, sleeplessness, or anxiety if they miss their daily walks.

Science shows us that we can "rewire" the brain to read faster, think more positively, focus more closely, or even become a better listener. We have the capacity to change behaviors as easily toward the positive as we do toward the negative. With repetition, these new behaviors and thoughts become the new you. But how do we achieve rewiring success? Based on input from a variety of respected sources, including *American Family Physician* (Zimmerman, Olsen, and Bosworth) and the *European Journal of Sociology* (Lally et al.), we have developed these secrets to changing behavior.

- **Understand why you want to change.** In the case of cancer prevention, you want to prevent cancer and the ill health caused by cancer. This motivation helps you implement and sustain changes in your lifestyle behaviors.

- **Have a plan.** Just the desire to change and the understanding about why you want to change is not enough. You must have a practical, easy-to-follow plan that guides your journey. Our Five to Thrive Plan provides you with the structure you need to develop your own health-promotion program.

- **Don't dwell on setbacks.** Why is it that we often give more power to the negative than the positive? If you eat healthy meals three days this week, focus on those days rather than dwelling on the four days you did not eat healthy foods. Dwelling on the negative simply reinforces those behaviors. Concentrate instead on even the smallest victories. Come up with a mental list of things you did well; think about what allowed you to be successful in those instances.

- **Avoid all-or-nothing thinking.** On some level, we have become an all-or-nothing society. Patience is not a modern virtue: we want it all, and we want it now. We also may obsess about doing everything perfectly right now, overnight, as if it's as easy as flipping a switch to instantly change everything—our diet, our workout routine, our relationships. To commit to changing your behavior is to accept the fact that it won't happen overnight.

- **Practice positive self-talk.** We could write an entire chapter on the power of positive thinking, but plenty of other great books already exist. Never underestimate the power of positive thinking. Visualize yourself being healthy, enjoying healthy food, exercising, and thriving! Surround yourself with positive, optimistic people who will reinforce and support your new healthy activities.

Following the Plan

We've all heard this phrase many times: the whole is greater than the sum of its parts. What began as a Gestalt psychological principal is now a mantra that is applied to business, families, and health. Throughout this book we too embrace this simple, yet powerful, principle when it comes to the five key pathways of the body and the Five to Thrive Plan. For example, the immune system is amazing and spectacular on its own, but when combined with other body systems, the whole body is nothing short of miraculous.

Consider using this book in the same manner. While you will hopefully glean great concepts and advice from within these pages on your own, you could potentially enhance your experience by sharing it with your family and friends. We encourage you to be creative and think of ways you can enhance the five core strategies (spirit, movement, diet, dietary supplements, and rejuvenation) in your life. Do this on your own, with a Thrive pal, or in a group of like-minded people. If belonging to a group isn't your thing, ask your spouse, partner, a family member, or a friend to read the book with you and periodically check in and exchange ideas and thoughts. This can make all the difference in your success. Some of life's great lessons and wisdom come from those who have experienced illness and regained their wellness—health secrets from the survivors! Learn from the survivors in your life and share your own survivor wisdom with others.

Remember that cancer is rarely black and white. There are gray areas in treatment as well as in risk reduction. Embracing the gray and setting expectations accordingly is critical. As with most aspects of life, wellness is a fluid process that ebbs and flows. Creating an ideal balance won't happen overnight, and it won't likely stay perfectly balanced all of the time. To ride the waves of uncertainty and challenge, we use the tried-and-true 80-20 rule. Try to do something health-promoting for each of the five key pathways at least 80 percent of the time. When you do this, you will be going a long way toward your goal of thriving after cancer. The 20 percent may represent those four days of the month when you didn't sleep as well, had dessert for breakfast, or sat at your desk for far too long without stretching. There is always another moment, another hour, and another day to refocus your attention on what it takes to help you thrive.

Meet the Body's Five Key Pathways

Cancer is very cunning. We need a prevention plan just as crafty and even more powerful than cancer itself. The key to cancer prevention involves training our cells to retain their optimal resistance and effectiveness over cancer while also creating an environment that is inhospitable to cancer growth. Cancer uses a multifaceted approach to survive—we need to do the same to prevent it. Focusing on one aspect of prevention is shortsighted and ineffective. It's not just one thing that causes cancer, and it's not just one thing that prevents it. This is where your body's five key pathways play a pivotal role. Although cancer can be daunting, the good news is that the human body is actually well equipped to fight it.

Understanding the body's key pathways allows us to prioritize actions that can help reduce cancer risk. We can positively influence our health through diet, lifestyle, and dietary supplements. Recent science, in particular the study of epigenetics and cell signal transduction (the various messaging paths inside each cell that translate signals from the cell surface to the nucleus, the cell's "command central," in order to create specific cellular activities), has shed much light on exactly how our diet and lifestyle impacts the health and function of our body.

Although cancer is ultimately a disease characterized by genetic mutations, the fact is that most cancers do not start with inherited genetic mutations. Instead, they develop over time because of mutated gene expression. Cancer promoter genes are turned on, while cell repair and cancer-suppressor genes are switched off. This aberrant gene expression changes cell behavior, causing cells to divide too quickly, to spread into the surrounding tissue, and to make proteins that call in new blood vessels. These changes, in turn, sustain the aberrant cells while maintaining a tissue environment that supports their continued growth. A few cells soon grow together into a colony of cells, ultimately forming a cancerous tumor, or in the case of cancers of the blood, they circulate in malignant cell clusters.

How does this imbalance happen? The food we eat, our activity level, a lack of nutrients, and even our emotional state all influence the behavior of our genes. Our lifestyle actually sends molecular messages to cell membranes that are then translated inside the cell and delivered to its very core, the nucleus, the home of DNA. There, these molecular signals interact with the DNA and become genetic switches that turn genes on and off. The on-and-off pattern determines the behavior of the cell and will ultimately move the cell toward improved function and health, or toward deviant behavior and disease. This scientific understanding has helped researchers and clinicians understand how and why lifestyle is such an important health factor. This leads us right back to the body's five key pathways—the superhighways of influence on DNA expression and the biggest determinants of health. Before we show you how to support the five key pathways, let's first take a look at the form and function of each one.

1. The Immune System

Many people who have had cancer believe that if they could just strengthen their immune system, they would be protected against further recurrence. Although there is some truth to this, creating a healthy immune system is not a matter of simply making it stronger. Rather than thinking of immunity as an impenetrable wall of defense that can be built higher and wider by adding more building blocks, instead, picture immunity as a troupe of sword-wielding samurais whose coordinated blur of constant activity creates a dynamic and agile defense. From this perspective, the best tactic for strengthening immunity lies in precisely fine-tuning the connections and the agility of the immune response.

When the immune system is functioning properly, it is complex and intricately choreographed, constantly adapting to our environment. The first step in this response is initiated by specialized white blood cells called macrophages (literally "big eaters") and dendritic cells (which process foreign substances). Macrophages and dendritic cells can be thought of as the samurai sentries of our immune system because they are constantly on the lookout for danger. Danger is spotted in the form of antigens, which are tags on mutated (cancerous) cells, infected cells, and foreign organisms themselves. Macrophage and dendritic immune cells recognize antigens and, in response, send out chemical alarm signals (called interleukins and cytokines) to call forth an immune response.

The initial responder to the alarm signals is the helper T cell, the battle strategist, which processes the signals and releases its own chemical messages (again interleukins and cytokines). The type of interleukins or cytokines secreted determines how the immune system will respond to the antigen-bearing cells. The response may involve stimulation of antibody-producing cells or it may stimulate direct cell-killing cells. The most effective defense against cancerous cells occurs when helper T cells secrete chemicals that activate killer T cells, also known as cytotoxic T cells, and natural killer (NK) cells. These cells are the master samauri; proficient and consummate killers. In response to this sequence of chemical messages, killer T cells and NK cells specifically target and kill the mutated cancer cells by injecting them with toxic compounds. This immune response is referred to as cytotoxic immunity.

As it turns out, many people diagnosed with cancer have impaired cytotoxic immunity. For these people, the solution for strengthening their immune response is specifically to *improve* their cytotoxic immunity. This can happen in two ways: by influencing the type of interleukins and cytokines secreted, and by directly stimulating the activity of cytotoxic T cells and natural killer cells. Seemingly simple things that we do consistently each day can directly enhance cytotoxic immunity. For example, the Five to Thrive Plan shows you how laughter, mindfulness, and eating a colorful diet can turn on the activity of cancer-killing NK cells and cytotoxic T cells.

The immune system is a complex, sophisticated example of the power of the human body. Supporting this internal defense system is incredibly important when it comes to preventing cancer and to thriving after cancer. Interconnected with the immune system is the process of inflammation. The inflammatory pathway is often misunderstood—and certainly underestimated—when it comes to its role in cancer progression and prevention.

2. Inflammation

A bump on the head will result in swelling and bruising. This is the body's inflammatory response in action. That bump on the head, a swollen joint, or an angry infection is inflammation. We rarely think of *cancer* as inflammation. However, research shows that an overactive, continual internal inflammatory response can directly contribute to the growth of cancer. The same samauri warriors of the immune system that kill antigenic cells also initiate inflammation. When you bump your head, white blood cells and antibodies are sent to the spot to help filter out bacteria and debris. A type of white blood cell known as a neutrophil will remove these foreign particles by eating them. This can take some time, so reinforcements in the form of macrophages often are sent to help clean up. Macrophages secrete a variety of chemical messages that create a multitude of actions. The immune messages direct blood vessels to bring needed nutrients to the area. This increased blood flow can cause tissues to puff up, which can then compress nerve endings. That's why sometimes we have pain associated with an inflammatory situation. Other chemical messages stimulate such cells as fibroblasts, the construction workers of the body, to lay down the scaffolding for new tissue. These messages also increase the rate of cell division so the tissue can knit itself together more quickly. When you see the redness and swelling of a bump or injury, think of all those hard-working cells in action.

In the case of a bump or cut, this is exactly the type of response we want from the inflammatory process. It's a surge of controlled activity allowing the body to wall off the injured area and rapidly repair the tissue. But what happens when, instead of a bump or bruise, the inflammatory process is initiated by more insidious and long-term injurious forces, such as exposure to environmental pollutants, stress signals from over-laden fat cells, oxidative stress, or even nutrient deficiencies? These persistent stressors can create an inflammatory cycle that continues well past the time of the acute exposure. This can, in turn, increase your cancer risk. The molecules of inflammation are designed to stimulate tissue repair by increasing cell growth and the flow of nutrients into the area. However, if the inflammation is long lasting and the rate of cell growth is too rapid for too long, there is more room for mistakes. These mistakes can result in changes in cellular metabolism and behavior, and ultimately will contribute to mutated gene expression—the hallmark of a cancerous cell. This abnormal cell, still under the influence of inflammation, will continue to divide rapidly, potentially culminating in the development of a tumor.

Although cancer growth can *result* from chronic inflammation, cancer can also *initiate* and perpetuate inflammation. When a mutated cell divides, it passes its mutations to the next generation of cells. Soon a little colony of mutated cells exists and each of the mutated cells in this colony bears unique antigens, causing the body to respond as it would to any other invading or foreign compound—with an inflammatory response. Thus, the growing tumor acts like an unhealed wound that continually triggers an inflammatory response, a response that perpetuates its own growth. Key genes and their associated messenger molecules of the inflammatory response are:

- Nuclear factor kappa B (NF-kB), often referred to as the master switch of inflammation

- Acute phase reactants such as homocysteine and C-reactive protein

- COX-2 and LOX enzymes, and their associated leukotrienes

- Such powerful cytokines as interleukin-1 (IL-1), interleukin-6 (IL-6), and interleukin-8 (IL-8)

Many of these important molecules of inflammation can be measured in the blood, and their levels can indicate the degree of inflammation that is present in the body.

Whether chronic inflammation is due to cancer or to other oxidative damage, it sustains cancer's growth. Thus, a significant factor in impeding cancer's growth lies in the body's ability to quench the inflammatory embers before they become a roaring fire. Inflammation is the body's call to action. If left unchecked, inflammation can contribute to a number of illnesses, including cancer, arthritis, dementia, diabetes, and heart disease. The longer the inflammation persists, the higher the risk becomes of developing these illnesses. Through the five core strategies (spirit, movement, diet, dietary supplements, and rejuvenation), the Five to Thrive Plan focuses on ways to proactively prevent and reverse internal inflammation. Diet, for example, has a huge influence on the expression of inflammatory genes. For instance, eating more colorful fruits and vegetables releases potent anti-inflammatory molecules, and diet is just one of many strategies to reduce inflammation.

So far we have discussed the importance of a well-coordinated immune system and a controlled inflammatory response; both pathways need the proper balance to function effectively. Another key bodily pathway with exquisitely fragile balance is the endocrine system, where hormonal harmony is paramount for optimal cancer prevention.

3. Hormonal Balance

The endocrine system is a major influencer of all other systems in the body. The glands of the endocrine system secrete hormones, which are powerful messenger molecules that help regulate major body systems and functions, including heart rate and blood pressure, energy production, wakefulness, blood sugar regulation, the development and function of reproductive organs, immunity, calcium uptake, and digestive function. We like to think of the endocrine system as a beautiful garment. What happens if you pull on a loose thread and keep pulling? The garment will unravel, right? The interconnectedness of the entire endocrine "garment" requires constant resetting and rebalancing. This interconnectedness also means that chronic internal stress on a portion of the endocrine system will have a profound unraveling effect on other body systems, such as immunity and digestion. The keys to the endocrine system are balance, rhythm, and homeostasis (maintaining that dynamic internal equilibrium). But how does hormonal balance relate to cancer prevention?

The link between hormones and cancer goes beyond the obvious hormone-dependent cancers such as estrogen-dependent breast cancer and ovarian cancer, or testosterone-driven prostate cancer. All cells, including cancer cells, have hormone receptors for a variety of hormones. No matter where the cell is located, it receives a message when the matching hormone attaches to the cell's receptor—and most often, that message is to grow and divide. Hormone receptors are intricate structures that form in specific shapes. Only certain messengers (hormones) can fit into these shapes, and once this fit occurs, the hormone receptor changes shape. A chain reaction occurs in the cell, ultimately sending a succession of signals all the way to the DNA.

This entire cascade of activity ultimately alters the behavior of the cell. Receptor-stimulated activity controls an enormous number of critical cellular functions. This is a good thing—for example, if the hormone calcitonin binds to its specific receptor on a bone cell, this causes the cell to usher calcium inside to strengthen the bone tissue. This can be problematic if it's a cancer cell with cortisol receptors on its surface that, when bound with the stress hormone cortisol, create an intracellular signal that increases the cell's growth rate. Unfortunately, many cancer cells have figured this out and rely on hormonally activated cell division. The majority of breast cancers are developed from cells that are studded with estrogen receptors and use estrogen to drive their growth. The cells comprising many solid cancers have numerous insulin receptors on their surfaces and use insulin (a hormone) to drive growth. Cancer cells also have receptors for stress hormones (cortisol, norepinephrine, and epinephrine), which, when bound by their corresponding stress hormone, cause increased cell invasiveness, increased growth, and even signal increased blood supply to the cancer cells.

In addition, these hormonally mediated growth signals interact with one another. For example, estrogen receptors cooperate with insulin receptors to create a combined influence on the behavior of DNA. The coiled helix of DNA contains our genes. Each gene is a set of instructions for a specific cellular function. When portions of the DNA helix unwind, the instructions contained in the exposed genes are read, or transcribed, into messages that build specific proteins to accomplish certain actions. In the case of estrogen and insulin receptors, when stimulated together, certain portions of the DNA unwind, and genes that code for proteins that stimulate cell division and invasion are activated. This is why estrogen and insulin are such potent drivers of cancer growth for cancer cells that have estrogen and insulin receptors.

The hormone cortisol also has significant impact on cancer risk. It is secreted as a part of the body's stress response. Chronic stress can chronically elevate cortisol, which can have serious health implications. When cortisol binds to cortisol receptors on a cancer cell's surface, its rate of cell replication will increase. Increased cortisol also results in an imbalanced immune and inflammatory response, in part, by increasing IL-6 production—a hallmark of increased inflammation. High cortisol levels also result in decreased natural killer cell activity. In fact, severe life stress may cause up to 50 percent reduction in NK cell activity by preventing the transcription of genes in NK cells that are necessary for cellular activity. Reduced NK cell activity leads to decreased immunity.

Hormonal balance helps our body work in concert. When we are healthy, our life is a wonderful melody, but when we are not well, we are out of tune and every off note impacts the entire orchestra's ability to perform. The Five to Thrive Plan shows you how to create hormonal harmony by using the five core strategies (spirit, movement, diet, dietary supplements, and rejuvenation).

The connections among the body's five key pathways continues further as we discuss insulin resistance. Insulin is a hormone that is secreted by the pancreas, an organ within the endocrine system. As we build our strong cancer-prevention foundation, the insulin resistance pathway becomes a critical part of that platform.

4. Insulin Resistance

To understand the link between cancer prevention and insulin resistance, we must first take a closer look at sugar, glucose metabolism, and how insulin works. The majority of dietary carbohydrates contain glucose. Sucrose (typically consumed as refined sugar but also present in fruit, some vegetables, and some seeds and nuts) and lactose (found in dairy products) contain glucose linked with one other sugar. Glucose in these sugars is easily absorbed. Upon absorption, glucose is either immediately used to make energy, especially in brain cells and red blood cells, or it is converted into glycogen and stored.

The pancreas releases two different hormones, one to supply the body's needs for glucose, and the other to avoid too much circulating glucose. These hormones are glucagon and insulin. If you have decreased blood glucose levels, glucagon is secreted to mobilize the stored glucose (glycogen) into the bloodstream. Glucagon also stimulates the body's liver cells to make glucose. On the other hand, if you have increased blood glucose levels, the pancreas secretes insulin. Insulin escorts glucose back into liver, muscle, and fat cells to decrease its levels in the blood. It is important to keep blood glucose levels within a normal range because if it drops too low, our cells won't have enough energy. If levels are too high, it can damage blood vessels, which can, over time, lead to a number of health problems common to diabetics.

When we eat a diet that contains minimal refined sugar, exercise regularly, and have sufficient vitamin and mineral intake, blood sugar levels can be properly maintained. But if the diet has too many simple sugars and refined carbohydrates, or if we skip meals, are under stress, lack sleep, and don't exercise, blood sugar levels will become elevated. The body manages this situation simply by increasing its production of insulin. The extra insulin matches the rise in blood sugar to efficiently transport the glucose into cells for storage and energy metabolism. However, over time, cells lose their ability to take in more glucose—a state characterized by insulin resistance. Essentially, cells shut their doors to glucose by preventing its chaperone (insulin) from entering. Both the insulin and the glucose are left to circulate in the bloodstream.

Cells then develop a strong need for the glucose that is barred from entering. In an effort to get glucose into cells, the pancreas secretes more insulin. Sadly, the receptors have not changed, and simply adding more insulin to the blood does not solve the problem. In fact, increased blood levels of insulin can create their own problems, particularly if there are cancer cells in the body. Simply put, insulin resistance feeds cancer. Cancer cells have huge requirements for glucose because they have inefficient metabolism, require rapid growth, and have higher energy needs to survive. Because of this, cancer cell membranes are loaded with insulin receptors. Even if some of the insulin receptors on cancer cells are resistant to glucose, there are so many insulin receptors that some will always be functional.

This means when healthy cells are insulin resistant, cancer cells can still bind insulin and bring glucose into the cell. And it gets worse: in addition to escorting glucose across the cell membrane, when insulin binds to insulin receptors, several other intracellular pathways such as insulin growth factor-1 (IGF-1) are activated. This creates a waterfall of signals that cascade into the nucleus, sending a combined message that activates the genes that signal cell growth and cell division. Some cancers rely almost exclusively on IGF-1 and insulin to stimulate their growth, and most cancers will use these molecules to spur their growth at least to some extent.

Because insulin resistance is such a strong driver of cancer growth, it is of paramount importance to reverse it. As you'll see later, this is one reason we recommend eliminating dietary refined sugar and simple carbohydrates found in refined grains. Removing these insulin-secretion triggers will lower blood insulin and IGF-1 levels. Regular exercise along with this diet adjustment supports healthy insulin receptors and is a powerful anticancer strategy.

You may be wondering about fruit intake. After all, most fruits are high in sugar, and yet they are still considered health-ful foods. Fruit does not need to be eliminated to address insulin resistance and cancer growth. That's because in its whole form, most fruit is packed with fiber, vitamins, minerals, enzymes, and polyphenols, which are important antioxidant and anti-inflammatory molecules that give the fruit its vibrant color.

This healthful combination of nutrients moderates the release of the fruit sugar, protects the blood vessels from potentially damaging effects of that sugar, and supports several other antiproliferative, pro-repair, and pro-apoptotic (cell death) effects in cancer cells. For example, a study featured in the *Journal of Nutrition* (Stull et al.) demonstrated that having a smoothie containing whole blueberries twice a day for six weeks significantly improved insulin sensitivity in obese individuals. In addition, active compounds in fruits and vegetables have been shown to enhance the activity of DNA repair and tumor suppressor genes, allowing these genes to slow cell division and facilitate cell suicide if the damage is too great to be repaired. To reduce the risk of many illnesses, we must break the cycle of constant insulin secretion and allow the body to manage and maintain healthy blood sugar levels. The good news is that through a combination of diet and lifestyle (specifically exercise), we can reverse insulin resistance.

The body's fifth and final key pathway is digestion and detoxification. Although this may seem like two separate pathways, digestion and detoxification work closely together and intimately rely on each other, so we treat them as one key pathway.

5. Digestion and Detoxification

Nearly every function of the human body requires nutrients. Where do the body's organs, tissues, and cells get their nutrition? From digesting the foods we eat. How do we protect our cells, tissues, and organs from damage? With detoxification. Digestion and detoxification together is the powerful one-two punch that both feeds our cells and protects them.

The digestive system begins in the mouth and ends with the anus, with a lot of activity in between. Starting with the saliva in your mouth—and including stomach acid, bile secreted from the gallbladder, pancreatic enzymes from the pancreas, and intestinal enzymes—food doesn't stand much of a chance in the digestive tract. It is mechanically and chemically broken down so the nutrients can be absorbed through the intestines while the food by-products are eliminated. It's also in the intestines where our immune cells, in concert with beneficial bacteria, sample food for disease-causing bacteria and other contaminants. About 70 percent of our immune cells live in the digestion pathway. These immune cells serve a critical barrier to the disease-causing microorganisms in our food. When the digestive system is healthy, so too is the immune system.

Healthy intestinal absorption is critical to get the nutrients we need while minimizing the absorption of harmful substances. Unfortunately, sometimes the lining of the intestines can become too permeable, allowing toxic particles to pass through the lining into the bloodstream, which can overwhelm the liver's capacity to detoxify these compounds. When the intestinal lining becomes too permeable, it's called leaky gut syndrome. Think of it like a food colander with holes that are too large. Using such a colander could cause the grapes you are washing to slip through and go right down the drain. What causes those "holes" to develop in the intestinal lining? There are several factors:

- Harmful bacterial overgrowth
- Inadequate digestion in the stomach
- Inflammatory intolerance of specific foods
- Free radical damage
- Certain medications, such as antibiotics

The good news is that the Five to Thrive Plan can help you avoid and even reverse leaky gut syndrome.

Optimal digestion and detoxification also requires a healthy liver. The liver is really "command central" because it breaks down harmful substances while activating and storing nutrients that can be used later. Compounds absorbed from the digestive tract are immediately taken to the liver. The liver serves an important detoxifying and protective role by screening these compounds for any that might cause cellular damage. Through the activity of hundreds of detoxification enzymes, the liver turns toxic compounds into harmless waste. These same enzymes are dual purpose because, in addition to detoxifying toxins, they can convert compounds into useful forms that the body can actually use. This is how we activate many of the vitamins, antioxidants, fats, and other nutrients contained in food into bioactive compounds that are used by our cells.

There are about a hundred different enzymes in the liver that carry out the complex process of detoxification. This group of enzymes is collectively known as cytochrome P450 (cP450). In phase I of detoxification, these enzymes modify toxins and pass them off to conjugating compounds, also found primarily in the liver. In phase II of detoxification, the toxins are bound, or conjugated, which renders them harmless so that they can be safely eliminated. If there is a problem with either of those two phases, toxic cancer-causing reactive molecules are released throughout the body and can damage cells and cellular DNA. That's why it's very important that both phases of liver detoxification are working optimally.

Health problems can occur if:

- Either system becomes impaired.

- There is an increase in exposure to environmental toxins.

- We eat a poor diet that is deficient in the nutrients required by cP450 enzymes or the conjugating compounds.

- We have an overgrowth of harmful intestinal bacteria that contributes to leaky gut syndrome and overwhelms detoxification.

Balanced enzyme activity is critical. Underactive cP450 enzymes will not effectively break down dietary and environmental toxins. On the other hand, it is also problematic if the activity of the cP450 enzymes outpaces the supply of the conjugating compounds used in phase II, because those new toxins are often more reactive and DNA-damaging than their parent compounds. Several factors contribute to overactive cP450 enzymes, including:

- Alcohol intake

- Smoking (including secondhand smoke)

- Some medications (acetaminophen and antiseizure medications, for example)

- Iron deficiency

- A high-protein diet

- Hydrocarbons formed during charcoal grilling

Conversely, there are factors that *decrease* cP450 activity, such as:

- Nutritional deficiencies, including protein deficiency

- Fasting

- A high-carbohydrate diet

- Grapefruit juice (specifically naringenin, which is found in grapefruit juice)

- Vitamin A or C deficiency

- Bacterial toxins

- The aging process

- Some medications (benzodiazepines, antihistamines, and cimetidine, for example)

The diet, lifestyle, and dietary supplement advice that is part of the five core strategies of the Five to Thrive cancer-prevention plan can help support proper balance between the two phases of detoxification. These five key pathways are the superhighways of influence within your internal landscape. How we support these pathways will determine whether we are to have a smooth journey or a bumpy ride.

Thrive Thought

John Muir, founder of the Sierra Club and perhaps this nation's most famous and influential conservationist, once said: "When one tugs at a single thing in Nature, he finds it is attached to the rest of the world." Thus it is with the five key pathways. This interconnectedness permeates the Five to Thrive Plan beginning with the body's pathways and ending with the connectedness we have to others. Embracing the interrelatedness of our health from a mind/body/spirit perspective and how our lives intersect with each other is the first step toward understanding what it takes to thrive. From there, everything just falls into place.

CHAPTER 1

Core Strategy #1:
Enhance Your Spirit

After one of our presentations on thriving after cancer, an elderly gentleman came up to us and said with surprise, "That was a very interesting talk." He continued: "Honestly, I sat in the back because I thought I might doze off a bit, which is what I typically do at these things." We laughed and almost in unison asked, "Why did you come?" He smiled broadly and pointed across the room at a woman talking to another woman. "That's my wife," he said. "We've been married for nearly thirty years. She had breast cancer more than five years ago, and she just loves coming to these things so I always go with her." That's love! Even though he anticipated taking an hourlong nap in a room full of strangers, this man had come anyway to support his wife. When he said "That's my wife," he stood a little taller, we noticed, and his chest broadened with pride. You could feel their connection even though they were on opposite sides of the room. It felt good, even to those of us witnessing it.

Mother Teresa once said: "Do not think that love in order to be genuine has to be extraordinary." Rather, the contrary is often true: a simple gesture, like attending a lecture, can show the one you love that she is supported and admired. By focusing on these simple gestures, we not only help transform our internal landscape, but we also lay the foundation for living a spirited life. It may seem odd to begin the Five to Thrive Plan with spirit and a conversation about love. Perhaps you were expecting us to kick things off with diet or exercise or even dietary supplements—a concrete subject you can really sink your teeth into. While all of those are also important—and we will get to them in due time— we begin with spirit because we firmly believe that only when you support your health from a spiritual place filled with love will you find success and thrive after cancer.

For us, thriving is achieving a sense of no-holds-barred, full-on release into the wonder of life. When this sense of exuberance permeates our being, we are compelled to live well. Exuberant living, even if felt as fleeting moments, is enough to sustain us on our path toward wellness. We deserve no less.

Eating a healthy diet, exercising every day, and taking all the right supplements may help prevent cancer. However, in the absence of a profound sense of the value of life, these actions will not grant us sustainable and joyful health and vitality. Health is, after all, more than the mere absence of disease. The Five to Thrive Plan advocates a program of health and prevention that is interwoven with a renewed love of life and desire to embrace our being completely.

Spirit and the Five Key Pathways

There is a connection between mind, body, and spirit. In fact, it is this interplay—the interconnectedness of all three—that can deeply influence the body's five key pathways. Here are a few examples of how each of the key pathways can be impacted by spirit.

The Immune System

Many studies have made the connection between enhanced immunity and feeling loved, joyful, hopeful. One study in 2009 (Dalmida et al.) found that HIV-positive women who had a higher spiritual well-being (and particularly those who engaged in activities such as reading spiritual material, meditation, and prayer) had less depression and higher counts of CD4 immune cells, signifying stronger immune function. Also, a 2007 review of eight studies (Marsland, Pressman, and Cohen) showed that positive emotions increase immunoglobulin A—an essential factor of a robust immune system.

Inflammation

Feeling empathy, compassion, and other positive emotions can also help reduce inflammation. A 2009 study (Pace et al.) showed that participants who were taught how to do a compassion meditation daily for six weeks actually had lower levels of stress-induced interleukin-6 levels, which is a key marker of inflammation. Another 2008 study (Steptoe et al.) showed that people with positive emotional traits had reduced levels of two important inflammatory markers: C-reactive protein and interleukin-6.

Hormonal Balance

Many studies show that our emotional state can impact hormones. In 2005, researchers (Steptoe, Wardle, and Marmot) showed a strong link between positive emotions and lower salivary cortisol (stress hormone) output. A 2012 randomized trial of seventy-one adults with a previous diagnosis of cancer (Bränström, Kvillemo, and Akerstedt) showed that a mindfulness-based stress-reduction program normalized cortisol levels within three months. This indicates that positive emotions and mindfulness improve the sensitivity and function of the hypothalamic-pituitary-adrenal axis—a vital hormonal system.

Insulin Resistance

The link between the body's spiritual and emotional well-being and insulin regulation has been documented in a number of studies. A 2012 study (Hartley et al.) looked at police officers, as policing is one of the most emotionally challenging occupations. This study correlated stress and depression with a significantly increased risk of insulin resistance, or metabolic syndrome. The more stress and depression that was reported, the higher the likelihood of developing insulin resistance. And, even more important, the converse is true. For instance, after a laughing episode, the study found, the activity of at least twenty-three genes that are involved in blood sugar control are altered for ninety minutes. The net result is better blood sugar control and reduced likelihood of developing insulin resistance.

Digestion and Detoxification

Many studies have linked emotions to digestive health. A 2012 study (Li et al.) showed an increased prevalence of depression and anxiety symptoms among gastrointestinal outpatients across China. Conversely, according to a 2012 randomized trial (Zernicke et al.), the symptoms of irritable bowel syndrome improve with mindfulness activities, as well as improvements in overall mood, quality of life, and enhanced spiritual well-being.

While the study of mind/body/spirit medicine is still a twinkle in the eyes of some of today's most forward thinkers, we ask this question: what if our thoughts *do* in fact play a significant role in how our bodies feel and how illness or wellness develops? One thing is for sure: there are no negative side effects from focusing on love, thinking positively, and being kind.

Physical health that is sustainable must begin in a positive place—a place inspired by love of life, love of yourself, and love of others. But this can be difficult when we are paralyzed by fear of cancer. For those of us who have seen firsthand what cancer can do, we understand the fear that accompanies it. Cancer is one of the most feared diseases of all time. But remember, our fear is actually an expression of our desire to live. Fear usually rears its head when we are confronting a situation that threatens to disrupt or destroy an aspect of our life. If we look *beyond* the fear, to what we are afraid of losing, we will discover that which we love and cherish. Thoughts of love infuse our life with spirit, meaning, joy, and peace. Thus, our fears become our moments of opportunity to live a spirited life.

Five Critical Action Steps

Spirited living is both the ultimate goal and an essential component of the Five to Thrive Plan. The "spirit" part focuses on five critical action steps:

1. Joy
2. Hope
3. Laughter
4. Service
5. Love

When our health and wellness are built on a spiritual foundation, we transcend the goal of merely preventing illness and move into the realm of living life with vitality—an expansive exuberance that permeates our existence on every level, not just the physical!

Joy

The first action step in the Five to Thrive spirit strategy is joy, or happiness. Were you born to be happy or unhappy? It was previously thought that our ability to be happy and experience joy was genetic. We were either hardwired for happiness or destined for doom. Not so! Modern scientific research, specifically the "science of happiness," has made some interesting discoveries. Happiness can be learned. Most people are in fact happy, and all people have the capacity to experience happiness. Happy people tend to experience more happiness. What else does this new "science of happiness" show us? People who are happier tend to be healthier and to live longer. In a 2005 review of several studies, Paul J. Hershberger, PhD, referred to a study that evaluated the autobiographies of 180 Catholic nuns and found that the nuns who wrote more positively lived significantly longer. Hershberger concluded: "Happy people have better quality of life, and research in the behavioral, social, and medical sciences is continuing to identify other benefits of happiness, including better health."

Preliminary research indicates that doing something very simple, like recognizing good things, is associated with greater joy and less depression. A published study (Emmons and McCullough) demonstrated that people who journaled about the things they were grateful for on a weekly basis felt both emotionally and physically better than those who recorded the hassles in their lives. This is an example of something very simple that we can all do. Even if we only do this every now and then, the benefits will be ongoing.

While the ultimate goal is to experience happiness and banish chronic fear, it is also important to make room for such emotions as sadness. "Happiness is not the absence of sadness," says David Spiegel, MD, medical director of the Center for Integrative Medicine at Stanford University School of Medicine. "Phony happiness is not good," he concludes, and we concur. People who consistently suppress sad emotions are basically teaching themselves to suppress other emotions as well, including happiness and joy. According to Spiegel, people who do not express their emotions have more of a tendency to become depressed or anxious. If sadness is your most genuine reaction to life events, then expressing this grief is the best way to interact with life. Although emotions are by their very nature temporary, they all deserve to see the light of day. That means that one of the secrets to experiencing joy is to not only express yourself but also *be* yourself.

Expressing yourself is living life with authenticity. Being authentic is being consistent with your thoughts, feelings, words, and actions. It means you are congruent with what you say and what you do and that you believe in both your words and your actions. If you sense that someone is being inauthentic, what are the feelings that arise? Perhaps it makes you feel untrusting, or you immediately discount the message and the messenger. In the business world there is a big push for "authentic leadership." The reason is simple: authenticity builds trust and openness and makes people feel more comfortable. Authentic living and experiencing joy go hand in hand. Unfortunately, many people live in ways that are not consistent with who they really are. Some try to live up to unrealistic expectations, even if those expectations are not their own. Going through the motions of relationships, work, and activities without our hearts fully engaged is living life on autopilot and leads us down a lonely, unfulfilling path.

You can practice authenticity by enlisting some help. Call on someone close to you to be your authentic witness and to inform you when she or he senses you are not being authentic. Choose someone you trust who will be tactful and gentle. Also, at the end of the day, think of times throughout the day when you may have been inauthentic. What would you have done or said differently to have been more authentic? Finally, as you consider your life, find the courage to ask yourself what parts of your life are simply just not you. What changes could you make to bring you—all of you—fully into your life?

Hope

One of the most important aspects of health, particularly in the face of a life-threatening illness such as cancer, is a sense of hope. This is why we have made it the second action step in the Five to Thrive spirit strategy. As the novelist Barbara Kingsolver wrote in her 1990 book *Animal Dreams*: "The very least you can do in your life is to figure out what you hope for. And the most you can do is live inside that hope. Not admire it from a distance but lie right in it, under its roof." Hope brings us motivation to engage in that which we believe will improve our lives. Hope is perhaps the most precious feeling that people who have faced their own mortality through an experience of illness have to sustain them. There is nothing that should ever attempt to rob someone of their hope—and, unfortunately, that happens all too often in the world of cancer. Restoration of hope is of paramount importance to people who have been diagnosed with cancer because it restores joy—and because it makes a difference to overall survival!

Hope increases the chances of long-term survival. This relationship has been demonstrated in several studies looking at the antitheses of hope—pessimism or hopelessness. A 2005 study (Watson et al.) determined that hopelessness in people diagnosed with breast cancer reduced survival at five years and up to ten years. There are many proposed mechanisms underlying the relationship between hopelessness and increased risk of premature death. Pessimism shortens the protective caps on the ends of chromosomes, the home of DNA in each of our cells. If these protective caps, or telomeres, shorten prematurely, the chromosomes become unstable. This chromosomal instability will either cause the cell to die or leave the DNA prone to mutations and cancer development. Thus, chronic pessimism destabilizes the chromosomes and ultimately causes the premature demise of cells or their mutation. Pessimism is also associated with higher levels of IL-6, an indicator of systemic inflammation and oxidative stress.

The converse is also true: optimism improves cancer prognosis. A 2006 study (DeMoor et al.) demonstrated that women with ovarian cancer undergoing chemotherapy who were more optimistic about the future had lower levels of distress, higher levels of perceived quality of life, and a greater decline in the CA-125 tumor marker test. CA-125 is a tumor marker used to assess increased activity of ovarian cancer. This study demonstrated that optimism impeded ovarian cancer growth.

Discarding pessimism and adopting a hopeful and optimistic outlook is a critical component to long-term health. It is important to differentiate hope from wishful thinking. Wishful thinking can feel like hope, but wishes do not take into account the reality of your present situation. Hope starts with a realistic assessment of the current situation and, based upon this assessment, creates two things. The first is the identification of the elements of the current situation that are undesirable and an idea of how these elements need to change. The second component of hope is a willingness to engage in actions to bring about the desired changes and to constantly reevaluate the impact of those actions on the desired outcome. This allows hope to remain tied to reality and facilitates new behaviors that are aligned with the hoped-for outcome. Leading a life based in hope will facilitate wellness and in turn support long-term survival in people who have been diagnosed with cancer.

Laughter

Jacob Schor, ND, FABNO, our good friend and colleague, believes that laughter is the best medicine. A naturopathic oncologist, he has written scientific papers on the subject and has even lectured to other health care professionals as to how they can incorporate laughter into their treatment protocols. Why is he so adamant? As Jacob says, you can't argue with the scientific literature, folks! In 2010 he wrote a literature review looking at studies involving the effects of laughter on allergic asthma, skin conditions, anxiety, depression, and even the immune system. His conclusion? "The scientific literature demonstrates that the effects of humor and laughter on health are far-ranging and numerous."

Perhaps the most fascinating aspect of laughter for us is the fact that it impacts us on a cellular level. Just the simple act of experiencing a big belly laugh can turn on certain genes and turn off other genes. Researchers (Hayashi and Murakami) found in 2009 that laughter improves blood glucose levels by modulating natural killer (NK) activity in diabetic patients. What was the research method? Funny videos. In one of their studies, they recruited people who were attending a diabetes management seminar. One day they watched funny videos and the other day they attended the educational seminar. Amazingly, just laughing at the comical videos turned on at least twenty-seven genes that then increased NK activity. This effect lasted for four hours after the video was over.

A 2005 literature review (Christie and Moore) summarized studies on laughter and immunity in people diagnosed with cancer and found that laughter stimulated a positive immune response, helped control pain and anxiety, and promoted general wellness. Based on their review of the scientific literature, the authors concluded that "humor can be an effective intervention that impacts the health and well-being of patients with cancer." Surprisingly, the act of laughing, even if you are not laughing at anything funny, improves mood and health. This has led to a new form of therapy called laughter therapy, which utilizes laughter as a therapeutic intervention. Laughter therapy has been studied in a variety of settings and has demonstrated positive effects on depression, insomnia, and sleep quality in the elderly; people with depression; and people diagnosed with cancer, among others. The key is to find ways to just laugh.

American poet and essayist e. e. cummings once wrote: "The most wasted of all days is one without laughter." Life is precious—let's not waste any more days!

Service

A few years ago we sat transfixed in the second row of an auditorium filled with more than nine hundred people, mostly health care professionals, as integrative health care icon Rachel Naomi Remen, MD, walked on stage. Her topic: integrating the spirit into health care. Her philosophy: fixing is the work of the ego, but service is the work of the soul. "When you help, you see life as weak. When you fix, you see life as broken. When you serve, you see life as whole," she explained. To live a spirited life is to value service. But what does it really mean to serve?

Abraham Maslow, PhD, famed psychology professor and one of the pioneers of the Human Potential Movement, once said that if all you have is a hammer, everything will begin to look like a nail. While Maslow wasn't talking about service, he was saying that it's important to broaden our view and look at things differently—this includes our perception of what it means to serve. The act of service can be accomplished in many different ways, and the best acts of service are unexpected, frequent, and heartfelt. Although we value the act of service in the form of volunteering, the idea of service goes beyond that initial definition. Service is more than something we do once a month or even once a week. Service is a frame of mind, a way of thinking, a way of being. Service is less about structure and more about substance—our substance as a human race—and how we conduct ourselves in every moment of every day.

To have a service mentality is to continually practice unexpected acts of kindness regardless of what you receive in return. For example, a nice gesture is serving your partner breakfast in bed on his birthday, but what would happen if you served him breakfast in bed unexpectedly on a random Saturday? And it's not just the act of serving him breakfast. What if you had a handwritten note on the tray and then enjoyed breakfast with him in bed as you told him how much you appreciated him? You see, service is not in just what we do; it's in what we say, and even what we think and feel. Seeing goodness in others and expressing that appreciation is an act of service that is priceless.

In the enlightening book *The Art of Possibility*, husband-and-wife team Rosamund and Benjamin Zander provide practical ways we can invite fulfillment into our human experience. The chapter "Being a Contribution" points out that life can be inspired from a place of contribution rather than the domain of success: "Naming oneself and others as a contribution produces a shift away from self-concern and engages us in a relationship with others that is an arena for making a difference." Not just making a difference, we would add, but *truly thriving* as you experience a vital and fulfilled life. How will you *be a contribution* today?

Rachel Remen says it so eloquently: "When we serve, we see the unborn wholeness in others; we collaborate with it and strengthen it. Others may then be able to see their wholeness for themselves for the first time."

Love

The fifth action step in the spirit strategy answers the fundamental question, "For the sake of what?" or "Why bother with all this?" We believe the answer is love and loving relationships. Several studies have demonstrated the health impacts of feelings of connectedness in people diagnosed with cancer. A 2005 study (Costanzo et al.) looking at women with advanced ovarian cancer found that the women who felt a sense of closeness and intimacy with a loved one (what the researchers called *social attachment*) had lower levels of IL-6, an inflammatory marker associated with cancer growth. Several studies have shown that people with certain advanced cancers (ovarian, breast, prostate, and other types) who have elevated IL-6 levels have a poorer prognosis. Together, this research demonstrates that social support and feeling loved can reduce internal inflammation and decrease cancer growth.

University of Houston research professor and renowned speaker Brené Brown, PhD, LMSW, says connection is important because it's how we are neurobiologically "wired." Connection is "what gives purpose and meaning to our lives. It's why we're here." In her acclaimed talk on the topic of vulnerability, Brown explained that in order for true connection to take place, we must let ourselves be seen. This is the essence of vulnerability. Perhaps you've thought of vulnerability as a negative, a sign of weakness, but nothing could be further from the truth. Vulnerability is the gateway to true connection and experiencing love.

Being in loving and caring relationships can actually strengthen your immune system. In the 1980s Harvard psychologists (McClelland, McClelland, and Kirchnit) found that immune function as measured by IgA, an important immunoglobulin secreted by immune cells, increased in students after they watched a video about Mother Teresa. This has since been referred to as the "Mother Teresa Effect." In the mid-1990s researchers from the Institute of HeartMath (Rein, Atkinson, and McCraty) had study participants intentionally feel compassion for a five-minute period. The participants had a 41 percent increase in IgA levels, showing a strengthening effect on the immune system. Enhanced immunity is supported by self-love, your love of others, and how you are cared for by those around you.

The Spirited Life

Self-improvement educator and author Stephen Covey wrote: "We are not human beings on a spiritual journey. We are spiritual beings on a human journey." We are deeply aware that we are more than a physical body. A spiritual life is one lived with acute awareness and genuine openness. Spirit is the fire in your belly, the life force that propels you into existence. Being attuned to the spirited side of life requires us to be present, engaged, and connected. Spirituality is personal and individual. For this reason, a hallmark of the spiritual Thriver is to be nonjudgmental of the spiritual practices of others. It is our right to embrace our spirituality, but it is not our right to judge the practices of others. The key is not to have the "right" spiritual practice; it is to be fully open to the fact that we are each a spiritual being. Embracing your spiritual nature will help instill in you a sense of peace, contentment, and fulfillment. And that's why spirit—which encompasses joy, hope, laughter, service, and love—is the first core strategy and the foundation of the Five to Thrive Plan.

Simple Steps to Live a More Spirited Life

Reconnecting with your spiritual self and leading your life with your heart can certainly be transformative. And, as with most transformations, it will take time and effort. Try out a few of these simple steps in your daily life to move forward—they will make a difference!

Encourage gratitude. Being grateful for others fills your heart with appreciation. You can encourage gratitude in your life by starting your day with thoughts of gratefulness. Before you even get out of bed, think of at least one thing, one situation, or one being that you are grateful for. Let yourself appreciate this focus of gratitude for a few moments. You could also keep a gratitude journal and each night before bed jot down the things you were grateful for that day.

Give yourself a glance of loving-kindness. Imagine that you catch a glimpse of yourself in a mirror. Smile at your reflection and acknowledge yourself, even if just for a brief moment, with genuine loving-kindness.

Speak from the heart. Think about someone you love and why you love them. Create some time to communicate with this person—either tell them in person or in writing about your love and appreciation. It doesn't have to be a big, drawn-out event—just a simple act of you speaking the truth of your experience of love and gratitude for the opportunity to share it. Be authentic in your expression.

Embrace favorite pastimes. What are some of the top things you love to do? Can you do at least one of these activities every day? Yesterday? Today? Relish the moments that you do get to enjoy these cherished activities, and if you can, insert at least one of them in each day.

Seek out social support. Don't underestimate the power of connection. If you don't have a strong support system with family and friends, consider joining a mutual-interest group, like a book club. Take a class or begin volunteering with others.

Cultivate laughter. Watch funny movies, hang out with funny friends, start laughing even if nothing is funny, and do whatever it takes to laugh frequently. The comedian Milton Berle once said: "Laughter is an instant vacation." Take one today!

CHAPTER 2

Core Strategy #2:
Let's Move

"*I know I should exercise more,*" a woman told us after one of our presentations on thriving after cancer. "But, you know, I'm just not the spandex type. Staying fit was never an issue for me, so I didn't really have to exercise. But now that I'm in my forties, everything has changed." It was pretty obvious that she was frustrated. And she was stuck with only one vision of exercise. Although we love what Jane Fonda, Olivia Newton John, and the '80s exercise movement did to promote physical activity, the hangover of that stereotype lingers. Many people have one view of exercise—tight-fitting clothes, mirrored rooms, and sweating on weight machines alongside Arnold Schwarzenegger lookalikes. In this chapter we deconstruct stereotypes about exercise and help you look at fitness through a new lens. In fact, let's not even call it exercise. Let's simply think of it as "movement."

Our bodies "talk" to us. If we sit for too long, lift a heavy object, or try out a new exercise, our bodies may speak the language of stiffness, achiness, or even pain. Yes, some movements can be uncomfortable, but the reality is that movement equals freedom; we are truly meant to move. Let's break this down into simple terms. In order for anything to be able to move, it requires the following:

- Rigid bar = our bones
- Fulcrum or hinge point = our joints
- Weight that is moved = our body
- Force or mechanical energy = our muscles

These required parts work in proportion to each other. If the weight becomes too heavy to be "moved," the rigid bars become too weak, the joints too stiff from disuse or disrepair, or the muscles too weak from inactivity, then we begin to lose vital mechanical energy. With the loss of this energy, we further compromise our ability to move, and we enter a vicious cycle of becoming sedentary for long periods of time. Henry Ford said: "Money is like an arm or a leg—use it or lose it." Just like using your money, you can use movement as an investment in your health. This chapter shows you how to earn big dividends so your health can prosper in the future.

Movement and the Five Key Pathways

The benefits of movement are far-reaching. We don't believe in magic bullets, but we feel movement is as close as you can get to one. Remember, one of the ways we prioritize diet, lifestyle activities, and dietary supplements is based on how many of the five key pathways are positively influenced. In the case of exercise, *all* of the body's pathways are significantly enhanced. Let's look at a few of the ways each system is buoyed by movement.

The Immune System

Several studies have shown that the strength of the immune system is directly influenced by physical activity. A small study conducted by researchers from the University of Nebraska Medical Center (Bilek et al.) showed that a twelve-week exercise program following chemotherapy significantly enhanced immunity. What was so important about this study was that it found that T cells, the direct cell-killing immune cells, were actually transformed into a more powerful type of T-cell. Lead researcher and physical therapist Laura Bilek said the research suggests that "with exercise, you might be getting rid of T-cells that aren't helpful and making room for T-cells that might be helpful." Regular exercise also increases the activity of natural killer cells (NK cells), which are critical immune weapons used to destroy cancer. In one clinical study (Fairey et al.) involving fifty-three postmenopausal breast cancer survivors, those who used a stationary bike three times a week for fifteen weeks had significant increases in the cytotoxic activity of their NK cells compared to the nonexercising control group.

Inflammation

Regular exercise is associated with lowered levels of several key blood-borne markers of chronic inflammation—namely high-sensitivity C-reactive protein (hs-CRP) and homocysteine. In a sixteen-week clinical trial (Arikawa et al.) with sixty-three sedentary individuals (sixty-five to ninety-five years old), forty-five minutes of aerobic exercise three times a week plus strength training using resistance bands three times weekly resulted in a 26 percent reduction of hs-CRP.

Hormonal Balance

While a single episode of exercise is associated with a transient increase in stress hormones, such as cortisol, regular exercise improves the sensitivity of the feedback loops that regulate the long-term production of stress hormones. This increases our adaptability to cope with stress and helps prevent abnormal stress-induced cortisol secretion. But exercise influences more than stress hormones. A 2010 study (Ağil et al.) showed that exercise helped ease menopausal symptoms in postmenopausal women. As an added benefit, the women reported improvements in psychological health and overall quality of life.

Insulin Resistance

Exercise can actually *reverse* insulin resistance. Some research (Ivy; Wallberg-Henriksson, Rincon, and Zierath) indicates that exercise is also the most potent strategy for *preventing* insulin resistance. Exercise is particularly effective at reducing insulin resistance in older adults. Clinical studies (Ryan) have demonstrated significant improvements in sugar metabolism with aerobic and/or resistance exercise training in middle-aged and older men and women. Exercise reduces the fat content of muscles, improves the tone of skeletal muscles, and increases blood flow—all of which decrease insulin resistance.

Digestion and Detoxification

Regular exercise improves all aspects of digestive function and is particularly effective at relieving constipation. Exercise also stimulates liver detoxification. Exercise's impact on the body's detoxification pathway is one of the reasons it is so important in cancer prevention. Regular exercise will decrease the activation of carcinogens (cancer-causing chemicals), specifically by enhancing the most important detoxification system: a super family of enzymes called cytochrome P450. Exercise also increases the body's ability to remove activated carcinogens by increasing the activity of important binding compounds such as glutathione-S-transferase that allow the body to safely excrete the toxins.

Because physical activity has such a profound effect on all five key pathways, it could be even more important to cancer prevention than diet. Let's take a look at the intriguing scientific research in this area.

Powerful Cancer Prevention

The American Cancer Society, the World Health Organization, the National Cancer Institute, and most respected leaders in the world of cancer prevention agree that physical activity can help prevent cancer. Why? Because scientific clinical studies have demonstrated that being physically active can reduce your risk of several cancers, including breast, colon, uterine, and prostate. What's more, exercise recommendations for those people going through treatment or survivors wanting to prevent a recurrence are shifting. In 2011, researchers (Davies, Batehup, and Thomas) stated: "Although rest is important in recovery from cancer treatment, there has traditionally been an overemphasis on conserving energy." More oncologists are realizing the significance of movement before, during, and after cancer.

The most compelling research associated with exercise and reduced risk involves breast, lung, prostate, uterine, and colon cancers. Research shows a strong correlation with the lack of exercise and increased risk of breast, colon, endometrial, kidney, esophageal, ovarian, rectal, and lung cancers. A comprehensive 2011 literature review (Wiggins and Simonavice) looked at studies completed over the past decade and concluded that physical activity can help prevent several cancers and can benefit people previously diagnosed by increasing aerobic capacity, improving physical functioning, and contributing to overall quality of life. The researchers also stated that some of the most common side effects associated with cancer treatment can be alleviated through exercise. Many studies demonstrate exercise's benefit on recovery from cancer treatment and on restoring fitness after cancer treatment.

If you've had a previous diagnosis of cancer and are working hard to prevent a recurrence like we are, you will most definitely benefit from increased physical activity. A 2011 report (Kenfield et al.) showed that men with a previous diagnosis of prostate cancer who were physically active had a significantly lower chance of dying of prostate cancer or any cancer. Those men who participated in vigorous activity (biking, tennis, jogging, swimming) for equal to or greater than three hours a week fared the best in terms of preventing a recurrence. A 2011 literature review (Davies, Batehup, and Thomas) concluded: "There is substantial evidence that physical activity can help relieve treatment-related symptoms, such as fatigue. However, there are now also promising data suggesting that physical activity after diagnosis is associated with improved survival."

One of our favorite studies involving physical activity involves breast cancer. In this 2008 study (Irwin et al.), women who walked briskly at least two to three hours every week in the year before they were diagnosed with breast cancer were 31 percent less likely to die of the disease than women who were inactive before their diagnosis. This study also showed that women who *increased* their physical activity after their diagnosis had a 45 percent lower risk of death when compared with women who were inactive both before and after diagnosis. Women who *decreased* their physical activity after their diagnosis had a fourfold greater risk of dying of cancer. Canadian research (Friedenreich) reports that the benefits of physical activity specific to breast cancer are likely associated with a broad spectrum of effects that include controlling hormonal activity, insulin resistance, and chronic inflammation. We couldn't agree more. With the additional exercise-derived impacts on maintaining healthy body weight, improved digestion and detoxification, and enhanced mental health, you can begin to see how powerfully healthy movement is.

The research we've summarized here is just the tip of the iceberg. The scientific data regarding the myriad benefits of exercise, including cancer risk reduction, continue to be revealed. Knowing that movement is good for you is the first step. The next step is to integrate regular physical activity into your daily life.

Your Fitness Foundation

What does it mean to be physically active? The American Cancer Society (ACS) refers to this as "intentional activities," meaning fitness that is done above and beyond routine daily actions like walking to your car in the parking lot or going up and down stairs in your home (although research indicates that these daily activities add up for better health). The ACS recommends that adults engage in at least thirty minutes of moderate to vigorous intentional activities at least five days a week. They note that forty-five to sixty minutes is preferred. But what is "moderate" and what is "vigorous"? Effort that is equal to a brisk walk is considered moderate. One way to know that you are walking briskly is if you are a bit breathless when you talk and have to catch your breath between sentences. Vigorous activities are generally defined as using large muscle groups, such as in the legs, causing an increased heart rate, producing deeper and faster breathing, and encouraging sweating. If you hear someone say "I worked up a good sweat today," she was likely engaged in vigorous physical activity. Another good way to gauge whether you are exercising vigorously is to measure your pulse (heart rate). If your pulse is at 75 percent of your target heart rate (calculated by subracting your age from 220 and then multiplying the result by 0.75) then you are engaged in vigorous activity.

Look at it this way: a casual bike ride to the store is moderate unless you are riding fast because you need an ingredient for dinner—then it becomes a vigorous workout as you race against time. Ballroom dancing is good moderate exercise, and doing the samba is good vigorous exercise. Mowing the lawn is usually moderate exercise, whereas digging, carrying, and hauling to create a whole new yard is vigorous exercise. As your fitness level increases, it is important to transition from moderate to vigorous activities so that the exercise continues to challenge you and, thereby, increase your fitness. Keep in mind, though, that the initial objective is to just get moving.

Five Critical Action Steps

Although your fitness program should be unique to your individual likes and level, there are five critical action steps that every physical fitness program should include:

1. Muscle strengthening
2. Aerobic activity
3. Stretching and flexibility
4. Proper timing
5. Optimal hydration

Muscle Strengthening

Did you know that every pound of muscle uses about six calories a day to sustain itself, whereas fat only burns about two calories a day? If you have more muscle, you will burn more calories and be better able to maintain a healthy weight. Muscle tone also helps prevent insulin resistance in the muscle itself, which is a primary source of insulin resistance systemically. Building muscle also increases our metabolism, which further helps us maintain healthy body weight and avoid insulin resistance. When we think of strengthening or building muscle, we may first think about weight lifting. This is an excellent way to condition muscles and is not reserved for bodybuilders alone. It is entirely appropriate for women to get just as comfortable in the free-weight part of the gym as men are. For people who would rather not work out with weights, however, there are many ways to condition muscles:

- Fast walking (you can wear ankle and wrist weights to build even more muscle)
- Jogging, running, or hiking
- Jumping rope
- Climbing stairs

- Doing push-ups or jumping jacks
- Using resistance bands
- Practicing yoga or Pilates

Weight-bearing exercises force the muscle to work against gravity or resistance. This action is what builds the muscle. Remember, when we energetically work large muscle groups like the ones in the legs, we are participating in "vigorous" activity, which is especially beneficial.

Aerobic Activity

Large muscle groups are also a significant part of aerobic activity, our second action step. To paraphrase the American College of Sports Medicine, aerobic exercise is an activity that uses large muscle groups, is done continuously, and is rhythmic in nature. The purpose of aerobic activity is to cause the heart and lungs to work harder than when we are at rest. Some of the more well-known aerobic activities are running, bicycling, and swimming; however, dancing, jumping rope, cross-country skiing, and in-line skating are also examples of aerobics exercise.

With consistent aerobic exercise, our bodies become conditioned, but if we don't vary the exercise, our muscles begin to lose some of that conditioning. If you've been doing the same type of aerobic activity, you could try to kick it up a notch. For example, if you are a brisk walker, try bursts of jogging for a few minutes during the course of your walk or hike. Inserting periods of more intense exercise within your normal workout is called interval training and greatly enhances your aerobic conditioning. You can also try an entirely different type of exercise class, or try the next level of aerobics classes.

Stretching and Flexibility

It is important to keep your joints limber and your muscles stretched. This is an important component of any fitness program, and it also helps prevent injury. Gentle stretching after your muscles are warmed up and then after you are done exercising is ideal. Stretches should not be painful but should exert a continuous and noticeable pull on your muscles. Some types of physical activities such as yoga or Pilates incorporate stretching into the exercising itself. In fact, yoga and Pilates incorporate strength, aerobics, and flexibility as a part of the routine. Being more physically flexible can make everyday tasks easier. In addition to enhancing flexibility, stretching improves balance, range of motion, and circulation. Stretching can also help relieve stress. Because stretching properly is crucial, keep these tips in mind:

- Stretching should not be painful, so don't force yourself while stretching; you should only feel mild tension.

- Stretching should be fluid and gentle; don't bounce or throw your body into a stretch.

- Don't hold your breath while stretching; use it as an opportunity to breathe freely and deeply.

- Stretch frequently throughout your day (in addition to stretching associated with exercise); also, stretch before you go to bed at night.

Proper Timing

The fourth action step is timing. Timing is everything, right? Actually, it's not *everything*, but it sure does mean a lot when it comes to physical activity. The first rule about fitness and timing is *frequency*. It is far better to do something more frequently (that is, daily, even if for short durations) than to just exercise once or twice a week or on the weekends (the so-called weekend warrior). In order for your fitness program to be sustainable and to confer maximal health benefits, you need to build it into your daily routine. Make exercise a habit. Schedule it just as you would a daily conference call.

The other aspect of timing is when in the day we exercise. Research has shown that people who exercise in the morning have a better chance of sustaining their activity in the long run.

Moving in the morning can also help rev up your metabolism for hours afterward as you begin your day. This can lead to quicker benefits from the exercise, which may explain why people who exercise in the morning tend to stick with it. If you can't exercise in the morning, just be sure not to exercise too late at night. In general, exercise helps with sleep, but if done too late in the evening, it can have the opposite effect and keep you awake.

Optimal Hydration

The average human body is 60 percent water. Water is essential to life, and yet the importance of it just doesn't get emphasized enough. Here are just some of the significant ways water functions in the body:

- It is used to make blood.
- The cerebrospinal fluid that nourishes the brain and nerves requires water.
- The fluid that cushions our joints is made from water.
- Water contributes to digestive juices and bile, which help us absorb fat.
- It is added to digestive waste products so they can be eliminated.
- It helps maintain our body temperature.
- It nourishes our cells.

Just how much water does the body need for all these important jobs? A common recommendation is to drink a minimum of eight cups of water each day, as most people naturally lose about eight to nine cups of water each day through sweat, urination, and breathing. Rehydrating ourselves with at least eight cups of water daily will help us preserve enough water to maintain essential functions. Another good way to ingest water is to consume foods with high water content. These include most fruits and vegetables. At the same time, coffee and alcohol are dehydrating. Thus, minimizing their consumption or at the very least adding extra water to compensate for their dehydrating effect is important. It is also vital to drink extra water on days that you exercise, as exercise depletes extra water through sweat and increased respiration.

While dehydration may conjure images of a barren desert and an isolated water mirage, it begins long before we feel parched. Even mild dehydration can slow your body's metabolism and even cause you to put on extra weight. On the other hand, increased consumption of water is associated with significant loss of body weight and fat. This has been demonstrated in several clinical studies of people who are overweight. The book *Water: The Foundation of Youth, Health, and Beauty*, by William Holloway and Herb Joiner-Bey, describes a study featuring 311 premenopausal, overweight (BMI 27–40) women twenty-five to fifty years old, randomly assigned to a weight-loss diet. The researchers found that the women who increased their drinking water to at least one liter (just over four cups) each day had an additional five pounds of weight loss over twelve months. The weight loss was attributed to an increase in metabolism (energy expenditure at rest). Merely increasing water intake helps you burn fat! Drinking water also prevents you from confusing hunger with thirst, so you won't eat as much. If you drink a glass of water before every meal or snack to help reduce the amount of calories you take in, it will also help you stay hydrated. If you want to get the most out of your fitness program—and the most out of your day, for that matter—stay hydrated. Be sure the water you drink is filtered or comes from a pure source. Water that has been filtered by reverse osmosis and/or active carbon filtration is ideal. Avoid unfiltered tap water, as it has been shown to have harmful chemicals and even potentially cancer-causing agents. Water in plastic bottles with the numbers 2, 4, and 5 are the safest, as the plastic is less apt to leach cancer-causing bisphenols into the water. Plastic water bottles with number 1 imprinted on the plastic can be used one time only. Bottles with the numbers 3, 6, and 7 should be avoided. However you drink your water, just be sure to drink sufficient amounts of it as part of your fitness program and your daily routine.

Getting Started

If you have been inactive for a while, please get some direction from your health care provider about starting a fitness program. Fitness trainers can also be helpful in creating a customized exercise program. Getting guidance early on in the process will ensure you are heading down the right path and will help you avoid frustration or, worse yet, an injury. If you are presently not exercising regularly, the most important thing to keep in mind is to start slowly. Baby steps are the way to go. This may mean that you start by taking a five-minute walk every day. Once that becomes relatively easy, increase it to a ten-minute walk. Eventually you can build up to three ten-minute walks daily. Over subsequent weeks, these short walks can be merged into one thirty-minute walk daily. This is just one example of how to ease into a regular exercise program. Set goals and allow yourself time to get there.

If you are ready and able to engage in more vigorous exercise, one of the best ways to start is by walking. Investing in a good pair of walking shoes and comfortable workout clothing is important. As you become more conditioned, add in weight-resistance training. We agree with the ACS and other experts that a pedometer (a device that counts your steps) is a good investment, as it allows you to see how many steps you currently take and then work to increase that number. Most pedometers take a little bit of setup, but you can get help from personnel in running stores or fitness trainers. It takes about two thousand steps to walk a mile. It's great if you can work up to ten thousand steps— or five miles—a day. Wearing a pedometer all day can be a fun way to stay active and to work toward a goal.

In addition to investing in a pedometer, we suggest you pay attention to *where* you are walking. We are big fans of doing as much exercise outdoors as possible. Studies show that exercising in nature—sometimes called "green exercise"—can have added benefits when compared with exercising indoors. A 2011 literature review (Thompson Coon et al.) asked the question: "Does participating in physical activity in outdoor natural environments have a greater effect on physical and mental well-being than physical activity indoors?" The answer? Yes, it does! After evaluating eleven studies including more than eight hundred adults, the researchers found that "exercising in natural environments was associated with greater feelings of revitalization and positive energy, decreases in tension, confusion, anger, and depression and increased energy."

Furthermore, the researchers found that people reported they were happier being physically active in nature and were more likely to repeat the activity. Although we understand that it's not always possible to get outside while you exercise, we encourage you to do so whenever you can.

Whether you are choosing a round of golf, a hike, yard work, or a dance class, be sure to incorporate the five critical action steps into your routine: muscle strengthening, aerobic activity, stretching and flexibility, proper timing, and optimal hydration.

"But I'm Too Busy to Exercise": Busting the Biggest Exercise Excuse Ever!

When we are busy, our fitness routine is often the first casualty of the day. This is ironic because exercise makes us more efficient and therefore less busy! Keeping a thirty-minute fitness appointment can dramatically increase the efficiency of your overall daily work and home life. In addition, exercise will help you sleep better! The bottom line: the busier you get, the more you need to get physical. You can't afford not to exercise if you want to keep up the hectic pace of your life.

Finding the Right Fit

One person's trash is another person's treasure, right? Such is the case with physical activity as well. What one person enjoys, another may not. A person with serious animal allergies, for example, may not choose horseback riding as his primary form of physical activity. Someone who doesn't care for country music may not choose a line-dancing class. At first, the only thing that may get you moving is understanding the benefits of exercise. This sort of motivation, while handy, typically wears itself out after a while. We need to be motivated to exercise because we enjoy it. There are many fun ways to move. Consider these options:

- Dancing to your favorite music
- Walking or running while listening to music or an e-book
- Hiking on your favorite trail
- Bicycling on a bike path through picturesque areas
- Joining a recreational sports team
- Exercising with a friend
- Taking an exercise class or working with a trainer
- Trying something different, like yoga or Tai Chi

Yoga is one of the fastest-growing forms of physical activity. There have been several scientific studies showing that yoga has significant health benefits. Yoga can be a great option for a lot of people. There are varying degrees of difficulty, so it can be easier to find a path that fits your specific needs. Those who practice yoga will tell you that it is more than mere movement. In Sanskrit (the ancient language of India, where yoga originated), *yoga* means "union." To most people who do yoga, it is the uniting of mind, body, and spirit. Yoga provides the opportunity to focus on mental and spiritual well-being as well as physical fitness. Although yoga is the practice of physical postures and poses, the focus is on breath, movement, and "being present."

Many of the studies involving yoga and cancer patients are small, but the results are compelling nonetheless. A 2009 randomized controlled trial (Vadiraja et al.) involving eighty-eight stage-II and -III breast cancer patients going through radiation therapy demonstrated that the women who participated in sixty minutes of yoga daily during the treatment had significantly fewer side effects (such as anxiety, fatigue, insomnia, and appetite loss) compared to the women who did not do yoga. A 2011 study (Bower, Garet, and Sternlieb) demonstrated that a twelve-week yoga program significantly improved fatigue, physical function, mood, and quality of life in breast cancer survivors. A 2004 study (Cohen et al.) featuring thirty-nine patients with lymphoma demonstrated a significant improvement in sleep quality and duration. Participants who did yoga (with 58 percent completing at least five sessions) also reported decreased use of sleep medication and overall better sleep quality.

Other forms of exercise that include a "mindfulness" component are Tai Chi, Pilates, and Qi Gong. Although these types of exercise are not as well studied as yoga is, they provide us with great exercise options. In particular, Tai Chi and Qi Gong are ideal for people who are looking for more gentle movements. A 2012 study (Fuzhong et al.) showed that people with Parkinson's disease not only improved their balance after doing Tai Chi for one hour twice a week for twenty-four weeks, but they also had improvement in bone and heart health, immunity, and mental health, and had an overall enhanced perception of their quality of life.

You may need to experiment until you find activities that you enjoy and even look forward to. For many people, variety is important. Doing different types of exercises will keep it interesting and help you avoid boredom that can develop from having to repeat the same exercise over and over. Exercising outdoors makes exercise more enjoyable, and people who exercise in a natural environment are more likely to exercise regularly. Exercise is movement, and movement should feel good on all levels—mental, emotional, and physical. Remember in chapter 1 when we discussed the importance of love, laughter, and joy? Well, this is the perfect time to incorporate more of that into your weekly routine. Choose physical activities that you love. We were meant to move. To deny that is to deny who we really are on the deepest cellular level.

Thrive Thought

Walk the dog! People who have companion animals—of any species—have greater psychological well-being than those without pets. This enhanced well-being increases activity level. The emotional support provided by companion animals and the impact that this support has on lifestyle, including exercise, underscores the important relationship between our feelings of well-being and our behaviors. Animals make us happy, help us stay active, and remind us of what is important. As the poet Samuel Butler said: "All of the animals except for man know that the principle business of life is to enjoy it."

Simple Steps to Get Moving

Try to integrate a few of these simple steps into your daily life— they'll make a profound difference in your health!

Move in ways you enjoy. How do you move now? What do you imagine you would like to do? What have you always wanted to try? It's important to make movement fun.

Track your fitness goals. Having goals and regularly checking in with those goals can help you stay motivated. Seek help from trainers and fitness experts if you are not sure what your goals should be. There are many smartphone apps and web-based programs that can help you develop goals and track your progress.

Create a routine. Commit to a regular time of day, every day, to exercise. Flexibility is important, but it isn't helpful when it comes to planning your exercise routine. Even if you have to adjust other things around your exercise time, it is worth it—*you* are worth it!

Start something . . . anything. If you haven't been physically active for a while, you may feel like a stalled car. But once you start pushing that car, it will build momentum and you won't have to work as hard to keep it moving. If you're lucky, your stalled car is at the top of a hill and your fitness routine will be off to a running start!

Know your strengths and limitations. Do an honest assessment of your fitness level and choose activities that match that level. You may need to consult with your doctor if you have not been physically active in a while. Set yourself up for success by creating a routine that is realistic and grows your fitness in small steps.

CHAPTER 3

Core Strategy #3:

Enrich Your Diet

Building a strong foundation with diet is absolutely critical to reducing cancer risk. Following treatment, there is often the desire to embark on a new, health-promoting dietary program, which is important and commendable. However, there may be a temptation to adopt more of an extreme diet. When evaluating which dietary program to follow, ask yourself this question: Is it sustainable? Remember, it may not be possible to make all of the necessary changes you need to make overnight, but if you adopt the concepts of the Five to Thrive Plan over time, you will soon be eating a health-promoting diet as a lifestyle, for the long haul.

Whether a person has had a previous cancer diagnosis or is trying to prevent cancer, we are often asked the same question: What should I eat? Implied in this question is the idea that there is one right answer. Although there are some universally accepted principles, diets must be individualized to be most effective. Dietary individualization can, and should, occur over a lengthy time period so that a diet becomes a part of who you are and how you express yourself in the world. As a rule, our bodies and our psyches don't respond well to abrupt and dramatic change. Even when cancer is the motivator, dietary changes typically need to be put into place sequentially, and relentlessly, to be effective. The Five to Thrive diet principles described in this chapter should be implemented with careful consideration and a high degree of patience. This will not only optimize your chance of success, but it will also give you time to get used to the diet and discover ways you can individualize it.

Diet is one of the most important components to thriving. Food is the vehicle for obtaining the nutrients our bodies need to function. What we eat, how much we eat, and the way we eat dramatically influence the nutrition our cells receive and, therefore, how our cells function. The health and vitality of our bodies, on a cellular level, is directly determined by the state of our nutrition. For that reason, diet is one of the most fundamental contributors to both health and disease.

Diet and the Five Key Pathways

As you may expect, diet significantly and profoundly influences each of the body's five pathways. Here are just a few examples of how diet directly impacts each pathway.

The Immune System

A goal in reducing risk of cancer is increasing the activity of central immune system cells such as natural killer and T cells. Many studies have shown that plant and marine omega-3 fatty acids enhance immune activity of these key cells. Other foods, such as mushrooms, have specific components that strengthen the immune system. Finally, we may not think of "good bacteria," also known as probiotics, as boosting the immune system, but studies have shown that such foods as yogurt that contain beneficial probiotics will enhance immune activity. A 2006 study (Nova et al.) showed that eating yogurt that contained *Lactobacillus bulgaricus* and *Streptococcus thermophiles* increased levels of CD4 and CD8 immune lymphocyte cells in anorexic adolescents who were immune-compromised.

Inflammation

Many foods, especially colorful fruits and vegetables, have been shown to reduce inflammation, thereby reducing risk of cancer. In a 2012 study (Ghavipour et al.), drinking just one glass of tomato juice every day for twenty days significantly reduced interleukin-8 and TNF-alpha, which are important inflammatory markers. In another 2012 study (Ganesan et al.) researchers showed that quercetin found in apples and onions not only reduced inflammation but also blocked the spread of the flu virus. Other animal and human studies have shown that quercetin can actually help reduce the risk of some cancers.

Hormonal Balance

One key to reducing risk of some cancers is reducing the amount of excess hormones, such as estrogen, in the bloodstream. The buildup of some hormones can increase the chances of developing certain cancers, including breast, ovarian, and prostate. A diet that emphasizes whole grains and fruits and vegetables has been shown in many clinical studies to reduce circulating levels of excess hormones such as estrogen. Many foods have antiestrogenic activity, including mushrooms. A 2006 review (Chen et al.) demonstrated that white button mushrooms were natural aromatase inhibitors. Aromatase converts adrenal steroid hormones in fat and tumor tissues into estrogen, which can increase the risk of developing some cancers.

Insulin Resistance

There are many ways to enhance insulin sensitivity and reverse insulin resistance through diet. Two key ways are to reduce intake of saturated fat and high-carbohydrate foods, which have a higher glycemic load. A 2012 study (Meyerhardt et al.) demonstrated that colon cancer survivors who were overweight and ate a high-carbohydrate diet had an 80 percent increased risk of experiencing a recurrence or death compared with participants who ate the lowest levels of carbohydrate intake. Even simple dietary habits, like eating more almonds, can impact insulin resistance by stabilizing blood sugar levels. A 2011 study (Cohen and Johnston) showed that an ounce of almonds in the morning helped diabetics reduce their blood sugar by 30 percent.

Digestion and Detoxification

Some foods can disrupt healthy digestion and detoxification, while many others can enhance it. Whole grains and fermented foods are two examples of foods that can enhance these pathways. Eating foods that are highly processed or foods that contain hormones, pesticides, and preservatives will put a strain on the detoxification system, so it's critical to reduce those foods as much as possible. Eating and drinking from plastic containers can also increase our exposure to harmful chemicals that put a strain on the liver and the entire detoxification system. In addition to eating whole grains and fermented foods, drinking green tea has been shown to reduce the risk of digestive cancers and can also enhance detoxification. Data published in 2012 (Nechuta et al.) showed that tea consumption reduced the risk of colon, stomach, and esophageal cancers in middle-aged and older Chinese women.

Diet and Cancer

We can scientifically make the link between diet and the health of all five key pathways. We can also make a direct connection between diet and cancer prevention or cancer progression. It is estimated that diet is responsible for 30 to 35 percent of all deaths from cancer. The higher the nutritional value of our diet, the more optimally our cells will function. This is particularly relevant when you consider that at any given moment, millions of cells are undergoing some form of either DNA damage or are battling the effects of epigenetic triggers that favor cancer development.

To combat this cellular stress, we rely on DNA repair and tumor suppressor genes. To perform their tasks effectively, these genes need nutrients. The job of these DNA repair and tumor suppressor genes is to provide the instructions to make proteins that do the actual cell repair and suppress abnormal cell activity and growth. Not only do we need the instructions to be correct, but we also need the proteins produced from these genes to be efficiently and accurately constructed. This construction process relies on a steady flow of nutrients.

It seems appropriate to use a food analogy when describing this process. Inside our cells, our genes can be thought of as floating in a biochemical and nutrient soup. The molecular flavor of this biochemical soup is dependent upon the compounds obtained from our diet. Just like a soup, all of the ingredients inside our cells interact with one another and combine together to create the final flavor. If we add more of an existing ingredient, or add a new ingredient, the flavor of the soup will change. It is the combination of nutrients that we absorb from our diet that interact with one another to influence the behavior of our genes and the proteins that they make. It is, therefore, the totality of our diet that has the greatest influence on our health—not one or two components. In addition, just as the flavor of soup becomes more pronounced the longer the ingredients simmer, it is also true that the effect of diet on cellular health and DNA expression takes years to manifest.

An increasing amount of scientific evidence is confirming that there is a very strong connection between diet and cancer risk reduction. A 2011 study (McCullough et al.) makes the case pretty convincingly. The study analyzed diet and lifestyle questionnaires completed by 111,966 nonsmoking men and women. After fourteen years, men and women with the highest compliance in maintaining a healthy body weight, eating a healthy diet that emphasized vegetable and fruit intake, limiting alcohol consumption, and exercising regularly had a 42 percent lower risk for death from all causes than those people who did not adhere to these healthy lifestyle habits. Risk for death from cancer specifically was 30 percent lower in men and 24 percent lower in women. The researchers concluded that a healthy diet and lifestyle that can be achieved in small steps over time does, in fact, lower the risk for cancer.

Five Critical Action Steps

The Five to Thrive Plan features five critical action steps you can take to create a fulfilling and healthful diet. The key to a cancer-prevention diet is one that is scientifically valid, is sustainable for a lifetime, and provides enjoyment. The steps for dietary action are:

1. Engage your senses.
2. Add more color.
3. Eat organic.
4. Eat more whole foods.
5. Spice it up.

Engage Your Senses

The first action step of the Five to Thrive diet strategy isn't necessarily about *what* we eat, it's about *how* we eat. The simple act of eating holds great health-promoting power if we allow it. In our fast-paced, modern culture, we've lost touch with the greater significance of eating. If you think about it, eating is one of the most sensual experiences human beings have. Eating involves all of our senses. We entice our appetite by smelling food. The visual appearance of our food can make us ravenous or can evaporate our desire to eat. We touch food, both with our hands and with our mouths; the texture of food can stimulate digestion and be an enjoyable part of the eating experience. And, of course, we taste our food, which plays a fundamental role in determining our food preferences.

Being aware of the way we engage all of our senses and taking our time to honor all aspects of the eating experience is often referred to as mindful eating. Mindfulness is a Buddhist concept that involves being present and aware of your surroundings in the moment. According to the July 6, 2011, issue of *Healthbeat*, published by Harvard Health: "A small yet growing body of research suggests that a slower, more thoughtful way of eating could help with weight problems and maybe steer some people away from processed food and unhealthy choices." The article further explains that this eating technique can even help reduce stress, gastrointestinal disorders, and blood pressure.

Mindfulness includes being aware of the smell, color, flavor, and texture of foods. James Gordon, MD, founder of the Center for Mind Body Medicine, said it best: "Mindful eating is what all eating should be." Mindfulness and engaging all five senses in the eating experience is a primary component of the Five to Thrive diet plan. One of the important implications of mindful and sensual eating is that it gives us the opportunity to feed ourselves with more than nutrients—to feed ourselves with nurturance. When we nurture ourselves, we eat with awareness. We consciously reinforce taking loving care of ourselves. Caring about our health and our bodies is perhaps one of the most significant ways to rejoice in the life force that we carry, which is sustained by the food we eat. We can't help but feel profoundly grateful with each bite of food, and gratitude is good for our DNA! The more gratitude we feel, the more stable our chromosomes— the home of our DNA—are. Stable chromosomes offer greater resistance to malignant damage, so even mindful eating is a direct cancer-prevention strategy.

If you are new to mindful eating, here is something to try during your next meal. Before you even begin the process of making your meal, take a deep breath. After you breathe in for four counts, think about the word "gratitude." As you breathe out for four counts, think about the word "joy." Now, begin to create your meal. Enjoy the changing smell, appearance, and texture of the meal as you prepare it, or wander into the kitchen if someone else is preparing the meal. Once the meal is ready, eat silently for the first several minutes, thinking about the food—how it looks, tastes, feels, and smells. For as much of the meal as you can, take small bites, rest your eating utensil between bites, and chew thoroughly. If you are eating with a companion, have a conversation about the food and what you are enjoying. When you are done with the meal, don't rise from the table quickly. Sit in silence and appreciate how your body feels, the flavors you still have in your mouth, and the feeling in your belly. Once again, breathe in deeply for four counts and think about how grateful you are. Breathe out for four counts and think about how joyful you feel. Now you are ready to get up from the table and take that feeling with you.

The sensuality of food is essential to our overall enjoyment of it, yet this is often the part of eating that our fast-paced culture causes us to neglect. How many times do we eat nondescript food out of a package that has no aroma and is bland in taste? Or people often fill up on foods with artificial, inflated tastes—foods that are high in fat, sodium, and sugar—thus dulling the senses. When we rely on these meals, we are missing out on the wonderfully varied qualities naturally found in real food. Unfortunately, processed and packaged meals have become the norm for too many people. Over time, with the repetition of this monotonous experience of food, it is a natural reaction to lose the joy, wonder, and pleasure—the sensuality—of eating. When eating is no longer a sensual experience, we lose a critical component of our diet—that of nourishing both body and soul.

The act of eating is one of the most significant and direct ways we nourish ourselves. Eating to nourish invokes health. Optimum health is built from appreciation for food and the ability to find pleasure in self-nourishment. Our hope is that people who are motivated to use diet as a tool to help achieve greater health and prevent cancer will, in the process, experience a renewed sense of excitement about eating. This excitement about eating is fundamentally an excitement about living. Feeding our bodies will only be satisfying when we are also feeding our spirit. Through diet we can regain our sense of engagement with life and in so doing honor and feed the life force within us.

One happy consequence of mindful eating is that you will have the opportunity to downsize your portions. Overeating—especially high-calorie, nutrient-poor foods—can lead to obesity, which is a primary risk factor for the development of most cancers. In fact, obesity is responsible for one out of every six deaths from cancer. While obesity is the result of a complex interaction of several factors, one of these is the quantity of food that we consume. Another reason that people eat more is that they don't feel satisfied or "filled up," so they continue to try to satisfy themselves with more food. It is believed to take about twenty minutes for the brain to register that the belly is full. If we eat too quickly, the feeling of fullness occurs long after we are truly full. If we eat more slowly, the brain has a chance to catch up with digestion and we are far less likely to overeat.

In addition to slowing down our eating, another way to reduce overconsumption is to institute portion control. Portion control is critical to a healthy cancer-preventative diet. Reducing portions will take time. If we reduce portions by half starting tomorrow, for example, it's likely we may not stick with it. In the days and weeks that follow, it's also likely that our portions would creep back up to where they started. Part of this is physiological. Our stomach increases its stretching capacity depending on the size of meals we eat. If we are in the habit of consuming large quantities of food, the stomach accommodates those meals. Over time, the stomach enlarges and hunger signals are generated if it is not adequately filled. Because we tend to eat when we are hungry, cutting portions in half or reducing portions too quickly will not allow the stomach to shrink and we will experience hunger signals—that familiar growl—that can be difficult to ignore. It is much more effective to gradually cut portion sizes and allow the body's physiology to change over time, rather than expect it to change overnight. If we reduce portion size over the course of a few weeks, our stomachs will shrink and eventually we will feel satisfied with less food.

Here are some tips to reducing portion sizes:

- Use smaller plates and bowls.
- Serve yourself 75 percent of what you think you want.
- When eating out, ask for smaller portions.
- Eat slowly, putting your eating utensil down between each bite. This will allow your stomach to fill up with less food.
- If you're dining out with a companion, suggest splitting an entrée.
- Drink a large glass of water before going back for more.
- Eat smaller meals more often to avoid becoming excessively hungry and bingeing.

As you implement these changes, your appreciation for the nutrients and nurturance that food provides will expand, but your waistline won't!

Add More Color

If you want to fill up on anything, we highly recommend filling up on colorful fruits and vegetables. As we like to say, color kills cancer! The second action step of the Five to Thrive diet plan is to eat a colorful diet—this is absolutely critical to both reducing your risk of cancer and improving your health. More than two hundred large population studies have shown that people who eat colorful fruits and vegetables are less likely to get cancer. Regular consumption of different colors and types of fruits and vegetables ensures an ongoing supply of a variety of nutrients that have potent anticancer actions. More than twenty-five thousand different cancer-fighting nutrients in plant-based foods have been identified. These nutrients represent a wide array of diverse compounds, including polyphenols, and in particular, flavonoids (a type of polyphenol). Flavonoids are pigmented compounds that give fruits and vegetables their vibrant color, but they also have powerful antioxidant, immune supportive, blood sugar balancing, hormone balancing, and anti-inflammatory actions when we eat them. Colorful fruits and vegetables positively impact all five key pathways that influence health.

The antioxidant action of flavonoids is an important reason why flavonoids are so healthful. Antioxidants neutralize reactive, or oxidative, compounds that are produced as a result of tissue damage from sunlight, radiation, infection, and chemicals as well as from metabolic processes such as breathing, eating, and moving. If our cells lack sufficient antioxidants, then these reactive compounds cause extensive cell and organ damage and ultimately disease. Our cells produce some of our antioxidants, and we obtain other antioxidants from foods—particularly fruits and vegetables. In fact, there are more than four thousand naturally occurring antioxidant flavonoids in fruits and vegetables. The protective effect of flavonoids against cancer has been demonstrated for all cancer types. These compounds modulate the activity of more than five hundred (and likely thousands of) genes, which in turn creates multiple and complex effects that cumulatively promote healthy cell growth and behavior, thus helping to prevent cancer development. According to a 2012 review article (Romagnolo and Selmin), intake of dietary flavonoids reduces the risk of head and neck, stomach, pancreatic, colorectal, liver, prostate, ovarian, uterine, bladder, breast, and lung cancers.

The scientific research involving compounds found in colorful foods and cancer prevention is not only fascinating, but it also is expanding significantly. An important study released in 2012 (Meadows) showed that a diet high in these colorful compounds is an important consideration for someone who has already been diagnosed with cancer. The researchers found that flavonoids inhibited cancer progression by activating tumor suppressor genes. Activation of these genes lowered the likelihood of metastasis (cancer spread).

An important 2012 review by Harvard researchers (Eliassen et al.) combined data from eight different clinical trials that included more than three thousand women with breast cancer and about four thousand women without breast cancer. They found that women who ate the most amount of carotenoids, which are cancer-fighting nutrients found in fruits and vegetables, had the lowest risk of developing cancer, especially cancers that have a poor prognosis and are hard to treat. Another study presented in 2012 (Steck et al.) at the 11th Annual AACR International Conference on Frontiers in Cancer Prevention Research showed that men who ate the most colorful fruits and vegetables have a 25 percent lower risk of developing aggressive prostate cancer when compared with men who ate the lowest amount of these foods. In this particular study, the flavonoids that showed the most benefit were citrus fruits, grapes, strawberries, onions, cooked greens, and tea.

Speaking of tea, several studies have demonstrated that the flavonoids found in green tea can help protect against cancer. Results from the Shanghai Women's Health Study (Nechuta) showed that women who drank two to three cups (these are small tea cups rather than large coffee mugs typically used in the United States) a day had a 21 percent reduced risk of developing digestive cancers. A 2012 research review (Kato et al.) looking at dozens of studies involving green tea and cancer found the following:

- Population studies show that drinking green tea can help reduce the risk of developing esophageal, gastric, pancreatic, prostate, breast, ovarian, and lung cancers.

- Human clinical trials show prevention benefits of green tea for prostate, breast, and lung cancers as well as for leukemia.

Colorful Food Menu

RED	PURPLE/BLUE	LIGHT GREEN	DARK GREEN
Apple	Purple asparagus	Green apple	Broccoli
Cherry	Blackberry	Avocado	Chard
Cranberry	Blueberry	Brussels sprout	Collard
Pomegranate	Purple cabbage	Cauliflower	Green bean
Red onion	Eggplant	Cabbage	Green pepper
Red pepper	Fig	Celery	Kale
Raspberry	Grape	Green onion	Spinach
Strawberry	Plum	Kiwi	
Tomato		Leek	
Watermelon		Lettuce	
		Lima bean	
		Lime	
		Okra	
		Pea	

YELLOW	ORANGE	BROWN
Banana	Cantaloupe	Beans
Corn	Carrot	Dates
Garlic	Mango	Grains
Lemon	Orange	Mushroom
Onion	Papaya	Nuts
Yellow pepper	Orange pepper	Pear
Pineapple	Squash	Potato
Yellow tomato	Sweet potato	
	Orange tomato	
	Yam	

Eat Organic

The third action step of the Five to Thrive diet strategy addresses the purity and quality of the foods we eat. One way to ensure you are eating the highest-quality foods is to eat organically grown and organically fed foods. Organic foods are produced without harmful chemicals such as commercial fertilizers and pesticides. In addition, organic foods do not contain synthetic substances that enhance color, flavor, or any other aspect of the food. Organic foods must meet specific regulations to be certified as organic. Many studies have shown that synthetic herbicides, pesticides, and fertilizers can contribute to the risk of developing cancer. In addition, these chemicals put a strain on the body's already stressed detoxification pathway, so avoiding these harmful substances whenever possible will help preserve our detoxification capacity.

Foods such as chicken, beef, and dairy products can also contain other contaminants that can stress the body's detoxification system and directly damage health. For example, a 2012 report (Nachman et al.) found arsenic residue in poultry products. The specific form of inorganic arsenic found in the tested poultry is used to make the chickens grow bigger and have more appealing skin tone. And yet it is a known cancer-causing substance. When the *New York Times* reporter asked one of the researchers what he does at home to avoid this problem, the researcher responded: "We buy organic." Eating organic chicken avoids this intentional arsenic contamination, and is one way to reduce your intake of pesticides, herbicides, and other synthetics. As you move up the food chain, these chemicals become even more concentrated, making commercially fed meat, eggs, or dairy significant sources of pesticides and toxic chemicals.

Emerging data show that organic fruits and vegetables frequently have the highest nutrient content, containing more health-promoting polyphenols, vitamins, and minerals than the conventionally grown alternative. At the 2009 Ecofarm Conference, Charles Benbrook, PhD, the chief scientist with the Organic Center, presented an evaluation of 236 studies that collectively demonstrated organic foods were nutritionally superior to conventionally grown foods 61 percent of the time. According to a paper published in 2010 (Crinnion), multiple studies confirm the information that Benbrook presented. Crinnion reported that in addition to having fewer toxic chemicals, organic foods had greater nutritional value—especially significantly greater levels of vitamin C, iron, magnesium, phosphorus, and antioxidant phytonutrients.

A 2012 review (Smith-Spangler et al.) found that antioxidant compounds, specifically the all-important flavonoids, were noticeably higher in organic versus conventionally grown produce. The study found that organically grown tomatoes had significantly higher antioxidant levels compared to tomatoes grown with synthetic fertilizers and pesticides. The researchers note that plants lose their natural defenses when chemicals are used in the growing process. It is the flavonoids and antioxidants that give plants their natural defenses; thus, organically grown plants will produce more of these compounds. This review also showed that organic milk and chicken had higher omega-3 fatty acid content compared with their nonorganic counterparts. Researchers also found that organic chicken and pork had 33 percent less risk of contamination with bacteria resistant to three or more antibiotics. A 2011 study (Brandt et al.) confirmed that organic fruits and vegetables had an average of 12 percent more nutrients than those that were conventionally grown.

Eat More Whole Foods

In addition to eating organic whenever possible, the fourth action step of the Five to Thrive diet strategy broadens food quality to include whole foods instead of processed foods. Processed foods are those that have been chemically altered in such a way as to increase the ability to mass-produce and preserve these foods. They have lower nutritional content and contain synthetic or chemical additives that are carcinogenic and put a strain on the body's detoxification pathway. How do you know if a food is highly processed? Look at the label, and if the ingredient list contains long, difficult-to-pronounce words, it's quite likely that the food is highly processed. The more "unnatural" the ingredients, the more likely the food will be harmful to your health. Whole foods are unprocessed or minimally processed foods, such as meat from organically fed, free-ranging animals; organic eggs; and of course, fruits and vegetables.

Whole grains are also a great example of a "whole" food. Such grains as whole wheat, brown rice, barley, millet, quinoa, and oats can all be eaten as unprocessed, or minimally processed, unrefined grains. In their unprocessed, whole form, these grains are rich sources of antioxidant compounds, fiber, vitamins, and minerals. Whole grain intake is associated with reduced risk of several cancers, including digestive tract, breast, ovarian, prostate, bladder, kidney, lymphoma, leukemia, and others. In large population studies, intake of whole grains has been shown to reduce the risk of cancer by as much as 70 percent. One of the reasons whole grains have such important cancer-prevention effects is because of their anti-inflammatory properties.

In a 2011 study (Villasenor et al.), fiber intake was found to reduce C-reactive protein (CRP), a marker of inflammation in breast cancer survivors. Women who consumed 15.5 grams a day of dietary insoluble fiber (fruit fiber, vegetable fiber, and cereal fiber) were 49 percent less likely to have elevated CRP. The researchers concluded that a diet high in fiber (close to 20 grams a day) is associated with lower concentrations of CRP and therefore decreased inflammation. A reduction in systemic inflammation increases the likelihood of long-term cancer-free survival. In another 2012 meta-analysis (Aune, Chan, and Greenwood), which is an examination of several studies, the intake of at least 25 grams of soluble fiber a day was found to be significantly correlated with lowered breast cancer risk. This study found that there was a relative reduction of 5 percent for every 10 grams of soluble fiber consumed. Soluble fiber includes seeds, legumes, oats, and bran.

Many of the chemical additives, food dyes, and preservatives found in packaged and processed foods are inflammatory and carcinogenic compounds associated with increased risk of cancer. Refined and processed foods are devoid of nutrients—meaning the calories they provide are "empty"—and they promote inflammation, suppress immune function, increase insulin resistance, increase the production of stress (pro-inflammatory) hormones, and can impair digestion and detoxification. There's no health benefit to refined foods.

One place that you are sure to find highly processed and unhealthy foods is a fast-food restaurant. In addition to using highly processed foods, these restaurants feature a lot of fried food options. High-heat frying (such as with French fries, chicken wings, and so on) creates substances called acrylamides, which are known to cause cancer. In our presentations on thriving after cancer we have a slide that reads: "If you have to drive through to get it, keep on driving!" We realize it may be difficult to avoid fast food entirely with today's hectic lifestyles; however, it's absolutely critical to reduce your consumption considerably. Start out slowly. For example, if you eat fast food three times a week, make a commitment to only go once a week, then every other week, and then only once a month. Trust us, you won't miss the drive-through line.

As you are weaning yourself off of fast food, be mindful of what you order at those restaurants. If you normally get a large soda pop, cut it back to a small, or even better, try water instead. Order the salad instead of fries, or get the grilled chicken instead of the fried fish. Or try a sub sandwich shop instead of a cheeseburger joint. Every little change you make gets you closer to your ultimate goal of avoiding processed, unhealthy foods entirely. At some point, you will experience a remarkable thing. As you move away from processed foods and start eating more whole foods, your taste and food cravings change. You will actually start to crave a bowl of kale salad and will salivate in anticipation of spooning a bite of brown rice and spicy black beans into your mouth.

Spice It Up

The fifth action step of the Five to Thrive diet strategy encourages you spice up your food. As previously mentioned, one of the ways you can enhance your eating experience is by tapping into your senses, and there is nothing more satisfying than the aroma and taste of colorful spices. Spices are a great source of polyphenols—health-promoting, cancer-fighting compounds. Polyphenols from spices (also found in berries, nuts, olive oil, and certain vegetables) exert powerful actions within our bodies. They can turn off NF-kappaB, a gene that is sometimes referred to as the "master switch of inflammation." Polyphenols also provide antioxidant effects, protect DNA against damage, improve the health of insulin receptors, thereby reducing insulin resistance, and positively influence many of the key hormonal pathways in the body. In addition, spices are flavorful, aromatic, and appealing to the eye.

Some of our favorite tasty anticancer spices include turmeric (curcumin), oregano, rosemary (carnosol), ginger, and garlic. You can add spices to the foods you cook or choose cuisine that already incorporates some of these spices. Thai and Indian food often have lots of turmeric, while the Mediterranean diet often has garlic, oregano, and rosemary. The scientific research on the active components found in some of these spices is substantial and growing. Perhaps one of the most studied spices related to cancer prevention and treatment is curcumin from the bright orange root of turmeric. In chapter 4 we describe this research in detail because curcumin is emerging as an important dietary supplement to lower cancer risk. It is one of the primary supplements in the Five to Thrive Plan. Curcumin can positively impact all of the body's five key pathways.

Garlic is another potent anticancer spice. According to the National Cancer Institute, "Preliminary studies suggest that garlic consumption may reduce the risk of developing several types of cancer, especially cancers of the gastrointestinal tract." Rosemary is a big part of the Mediterranean diet—one of the most scientifically valid cancer-prevention and health-promoting diets out there. The active compound in rosemary is carnosol. A 2011 review (Johnson) described several cellular test tube studies showing carnosol's anticancer activity against prostate, breast, and skin cancer cells as well as three different leukemia cell lines.

A 2011 small clinical trial (Zick et al.) demonstrated that participants at high risk for colorectal cancer who ate ginger root had lower levels of colon inflammatory markers compared with participants who took the placebo. The researchers concluded that ginger has potential to help reduce risk of colon cancer. A 2009 literature review (Aggarwal et al.) evaluated forty-one common dietary spices and concluded that "many of the spices mentioned in this article have been regarded in a variety of cultures as having health benefits for centuries, such as garlic and ginger. Overall our review suggests 'adding spice to your life' may serve as a healthy and delicious way to ward off cancer and other chronic diseases." For some great-tasting and health-promoting recipes, see the books listed in the Resources.

Getting Started

For optimum cancer prevention, we recommend the following daily serving guidelines: 5 to 10 servings of fruits and vegetables, 4 servings of seeds/nuts/healthy oils, 3 to 6 servings of whole grains, 2 to 3 servings of protein, and up to 2 ounces of dark chocolate. Are you thinking it may be impossible to get that many recommended servings of fruits and vegetables? It may be easier than you think. First, let's start with what "a serving" actually is:

- Vegetables = 1 cup of raw or leafy greens; $^1/_2$ cup of raw nonleafy vegetables; $^1/_2$ cup of cooked vegetables; $^1/_2$ cup of fresh vegetable juice

- Fruit = 1 medium fruit; $^1/_2$ cup cut-up fruit; 1 cup berries; 4 ounces 100 percent fresh juice; $^1/_4$ cup dried fruit

- Seeds or nuts = $^1/_4$ cup

- Healthy oils such as olive = 1 tablespoon

- Whole grains = 1 slice of whole wheat, rye, or other whole-grain bread; $^1/_2$ cup whole-grain cereal; $^1/_2$ cup cooked whole-kernel corn; 1 small ear of corn; $^1/_2$ cup cooked whole-grain pasta

- Beans (legumes) = $^1/_2$ cup cooked
- Protein = 3 to 4 ounces (size of a deck of cards) of grass-fed meat, deep-sea fish or shellfish, or organic tofu

Consider the following meal plans:

	MEALS	FOOD	APPROXIMATE SERVINGS
Day 1	Breakfast	Oatmeal with blueberries, raw almonds, and agave nectar	3 servings fruit 5 servings vegetables 2 serving nuts 3–5 servings whole grains 3 servings protein
	Lunch	A large bowl of mixed vegetable salad with a grilled chicken breast and olive oil–based salad dressing	
	Dinner	Tofu, mushroom, onion, cashew, ginger, garlic stir-fry in olive oil with brown rice	
	Snacks	Apple, trail mix, 2 ounces dark chocolate	
Day 2	Breakfast	Fresh fruit, flaxseed meal, and protein powder shake	3 servings fruit 6 servings vegetables 1 serving seeds 4 servings whole grains 4 servings protein
	Lunch	Egg salad, lettuce, and tomato sandwich on whole wheat bread with vegetable soup	
	Dinner	Chicken and mixed vegetable coconut milk curry over quinoa	
	Snacks	Tortilla chips and guacamole	
Day 3	Breakfast	2 hard-boiled eggs, whole-grain toast, and an orange	2 servings fruit 5 servings vegetables 2 servings legumes 4 servings whole grains 3 servings protein
	Lunch	Black beans and rice with a side of steamed kale	
	Dinner	Halibut, asparagus, and sweet potato	
	Snacks	Strawberries with dark chocolate sauce	

Frequently Asked Questions

Questions about diet are definitely the most common questions that we are asked. Typically questions fit into two categories: things to avoid and special diets. Here's a rundown of our thoughts (and the latest science) on soy, alcohol, caffeine/coffee, dairy, eggs, sugar, chocolate, and Bisphenol A (BPA). We also discuss vegetarian, alkaline, food allergy elimination, wheat-free, and detoxification diets.

Should I Avoid Soy?

Soy foods and the isoflavones they contain have been shown in many studies to be potent anticancer compounds. In populations in which soy intake is a main part of the diet, such as in many Asian countries, the incidence of most cancers is lower than in populations that don't consume soy. Furthermore, when people from those Asian countries move to Western countries and adopt a Western diet that has little to no soy, their rates of cancer increase to the same rates of their Western counterparts. Epidemiological studies have shown that soy consumption can reduce the risk of developing various cancers, including cancers of the prostate and breast.

Despite this data, however, many women have been instructed to avoid soy if they have a history of estrogen receptor positive (ER+) breast cancer. This is because soy contains compounds known as phytoestrogens that can bind to estrogen receptors and could therefore theoretically stimulate those estrogen receptors much in the same way that estrogen does, thereby accelerating the growth of estrogen-dependent cancers. However, there are two major types of estrogen receptors, and soy preferentially binds to the sub-type beta estrogen receptor, which, when activated, inhibits the cancer growth–promoting sub-type alpha estrogen receptor. While this may seem confusing, several clinical trials of women with a history of breast cancer have demonstrated that soy protein intake is, in fact, associated with a *decreased* risk of recurrence and a *decreased* risk of dying from breast cancer—even ER+ breast cancer. This decreased risk of cancer recurrence and death due to soy is evident in women receiving tamoxifen therapy, a known estrogen receptor–blocking agent, as well as in women not taking tamoxifen.

The protective effect of soy is demonstrated in both menopausal and premenopausal women. The cancer-prevention effect of soy in women with a history of breast cancer was studied in an analysis of four large epidemiological trials (S. J. Nechuta et al.). After an average of seven years following their breast cancer diagnosis, women who ate more than 23 milligrams of soy per day (the equivalent of one glass of soy milk or one-half cup of tofu), providing 10 milligrams of soy isoflavones, lowered their risk of dying from breast cancer by 17 percent and reduced their risk for breast cancer recurrence by 15 percent, compared to women who consumed 0.48 milligrams of soy per day or less.

Although the anticancer mechanism of soy is not fully understood, there are several well-evidenced theories. The isoflavones in soy slow the growth rate of cancer cells, have strong antioxidant effects, and reduce inflammation. Clinical trials indicate that soy consumption is associated with a decreased risk of cancers, including breast cancer, even in women with a history of ER+ breast cancer. Whole soy foods such as tofu, soy milk, edamame, and soy flour are associated with this preventive benefit. Isolated soy protein, found in snack bars or powders, lacks the beneficial isoflavones found in whole soy foods and is therefore not as beneficial.

Should I Avoid Alcohol?

Many of us enjoy the pleasures of a glass of wine, a cocktail, or a beer. But drinking alcohol can be confusing to those with cancer, those with a history of cancer, or people trying to prevent cancer. Given the link between excess alcohol consumption and an increased risk of cancer, it's a valid concern. In a prospective study of more than 350,000 adults (Schutz et al.), about 10 percent of all cancer in European men and 3 percent of all cancer in European women could be the result of current and former alcohol consumption. Cancers of the upper digestive tract (especially in men), liver cancer, and breast cancer in women are most attributable to alcohol intake.

The majority of this risk is associated with moderate alcohol consumption, defined as more than two daily drinks for men or one daily drink for women. Greater than moderate alcohol consumption is causally related to cancers of the breast, colon, mouth, throat, esophagus, and liver, and the risk for all cancers increases with additional daily drinking. This means that there is a direct and linear relationship between the quantity of alcohol consumed over one's lifetime and the risk of cancer. In some situations, any alcohol consumption is problematic. For instance, in postmenopausal women who have a history of breast cancer, any regular alcohol consumption of more than one drink daily, of any type, increases the risk of breast cancer recurrence. In a 2011 prospective study (Wendy et al.), 105,986 women were followed for several decades. The researchers found that having three to six glasses of wine a week raised a woman's risk of breast cancer by 15 percent. The effects were cumulative: with each additional glass above the six weekly glasses, there was an additional 10 percent risk. While such an increase may sound alarming, this risk actually translates into only a very small actual risk for the average woman. For instance, an average fifty-year-old woman has about a 3 percent risk of developing breast cancer over the next five years of her life. If this woman consumed three to six glasses of wine each week, she would increase this risk by 15 percent, which would increase her risk to 3.45 percent.

The studies on alcohol consumption and risk rely on self-reports, which are notorious for underreporting actual consumption, so the risk may be exaggerated. In addition, studies conducted to date have not been able to determine if changing one's alcohol consumption from more to less (or vice versa) over time changes the risk. The bottom line? A recent editorial (Narod) pointed out that based on the findings, women who consumed two or more drinks a day would see their ten-year risk of breast cancer climb to 4.1 percent from 2.8 percent. And for women who had one drink a day, it would rise to 3.5 percent from 2.8 percent.

Interestingly, there is an emerging body of research about the health *benefits* of moderate red wine consumption. "Moderate consumption" is defined as no more than one glass daily for women and up to two glasses daily for men. Red wine contains more than twenty different polyphenols, which are compounds that have potent antioxidant capacity, stimulate repair of damaged cells, reduce blood stickiness, stimulate the transport of cholesterol away from blood vessels to the liver for processing, reduce insulin resistance, and interrupt chronic inflammatory responses. Polyphenols are powerful compounds.

White wine only contains 10 percent of the polyphenols of red wine because the polyphenols are primarily derived from the dark-pigmented compounds in grape skins. The greatest polyphenol content is found in red wine made from grapes exposed to significant sunlight and then macerated in oak barrels for the longest period of time. The oak tannins from the barrels add to the polyphenols, so red wine aged in oak barrels not only tastes good but is also healthier. And, of course, wine made from organically grown grapes avoids synthetic pesticides. According to the scientific literature, one daily glass of red wine reduces elevated blood sugar, is correlated with better weight control, and reduces inflammation—all of which are important cancer-prevention strategies.

What is the bottom line on alcohol? If you don't drink now, don't start. If you do drink, be aware of the risk, determine your comfort level with that risk, and make your decisions accordingly.

Should I Avoid Caffeine/Coffee?

Some caffeinated beverages, such as coffee and tea, are not associated with increased cancer risk. In fact, coffee and tea are rich sources of polyphenols, contain powerful antioxidants, protect DNA, and have anti-inflammatory effects. Other caffeinated beverages, such as caffeinated soda, are not beneficial and are, in fact, harmful. Most soda pops have chemical additives and contain either lots of sugar or potentially cancer-causing sugar substitutes. Although caffeine is not, in and of itself, cancer-causing, drinking excess caffeine will compromise the stress response and over time can contribute to excess cortisol. Elevated cortisol suppresses the immune system and is associated with increased inflammation, insulin resistance, and risk of cancer progression.

Having one to two cups of coffee or black or green tea a day is unlikely to cause harm and provides some protective effects for most cancers. A 2011 review (Yu et al.) showed that coffee consumption slightly reduced total cancer incidence. Another review (Shafique et al.) demonstrated that those who consumed more than three cups of coffee daily reduced the risk of developing aggressive prostate cancer by 55 percent compared to noncoffee drinkers. One type of cancer that showed a mixed response to caffeine is lung cancer. A 2012 meta-analysis (Wang et al.) found that increased consumption of green tea, which contains small amounts of caffeine, lowered the relative risk of lung cancer by 18 percent for every two cups consumed on a daily basis. However, the same meta-analysis found that drinking two cups of coffee every day increased the relative risk of developing lung cancer by 14 percent. In contrast, coffee drinking lowers the risk of liver cancer (Sang et al.), colon cancer (Li et al.), pancreatic cancer (Dong, Zou, and Yu), and uterine cancer (Je and Giovannucci). As for other types of cancer, coffee doesn't appear to raise or lower risk. Thus, aside from individuals with other risk factors for lung cancer, such as cigarette smoking, coffee drinking appears to be beneficial, or at least neutral, to the risk of developing cancer.

For those coffee drinkers out there, one important thing that you can do to lower any potential risk from coffee is to consume coffee made from organically grown coffee beans. The process of coffee preparation, which relies on combining coffee beans with hot water, extracts cancer-causing pesticides; using organic coffee beans avoids this exposure. Furthermore, if you consume decaffeinated coffee, opt for water-processed decaf that removes the caffeine without the use of harsh chemicals.

Should I Avoid Dairy?

Generally speaking, excessive reliance on dairy for calories, protein, or other nutrients is ill advised. Dairy is a source of saturated fat, and nonorganic dairy products contain residual antibiotics, hormones, and pesticides. Increased dairy consumption ups the risk of certain cancers, such as ovarian and prostate. On the flip side, dairy is a rich source of certain cancer-preventive compounds—namely, conjugated linoleic acid (CLA) and vitamin K_2. CLA has been demonstrated in several preclinical studies to increase cancer cell death. There appears to be a modest reduction of breast cancer risk with consumption of low-fat dairy.

Dairy products, in particular butter, are rich sources of CLA. This is not to say we should be eating large amounts of butter, however. Vitamin K_2 is an important vitamin in the control of angiogenesis, or the development of new blood vessels. As a tumor grows, it requires blood supply to keep growing. Inhibiting angiogenesis is a critical part of our internal defense against tumor growth. Dairy products, particularly cheese, are a rich source of vitamin K_2, lending cheese a modest protective effect. If you decide to include dairy in your diet, it is very important that it be organic. It is important to note that the majority of vitamin K_2 in our bodies is derived from the bacterial breakdown of foods in our digestive tract. Therefore, a better way to ensure adequate vitamin K_2 is to make sure our digestive tracts contain sufficient beneficial bacteria. This can be accomplished by eating fermented foods—such as yogurt (be sure it is natural, with low sugar content), sauerkraut, and kefir—or taking a probiotic supplement every day.

Should I Avoid Eggs?

The scientific data on the relationship between egg consumption and cancer risk is mixed. Some studies suggest that high intake of eggs is associated with an increased risk of certain cancers—namely, ovarian, colon, and some other cancers of the digestive tract. However, other studies have failed to find this association. Until this association is further clarified, it may be appropriate for people at higher risk for ovarian and colon cancer to limit egg intake to fewer than five eggs a week. It is also important to prepare eggs in a manner that avoids oxidizing their fats. The best methods of egg preparation are boiling and poaching. Frying and scrambling eggs denatures their cholesterol and fats, making these potentially deleterious to our health. If you do consume eggs, we suggest that you eat eggs from free-range, organically fed chickens—or even better—from the farm of your local organic farmer. These eggs are more nutritious, have a better ratio of anti-inflammatory fats, and come from healthier and happier chickens!

Should I Avoid Sugar?

All the cells in the body rely on sugar to make energy, including cancer cells. Cancer cells are very inefficient at metabolizing sugar into energy; they feed themselves differently than do normal cells. Cancer cells make energy (ATP) from sugar (glucose) via a process called glycolysis. Normal cells combine glucose with oxygen in a very efficient process known as oxidative phosphorylation, which makes thirty-four molecules of ATP from one molecule of glucose. Glycolysis, used by tumor cells, only generates two molecules of ATP from each molecule of glucose. Why would cancers preferentially use glycolysis, such an inefficient process? It seems that glycolysis, while generating less energy, has the advantage of also making the building blocks for DNA, protein, and lipid molecules—all of which are essential to supporting the growth of rapidly dividing cancer cells. Also, glycolysis lowers the pH of the tissue around the cancer cell, which causes normal cells to die and blood vessels to develop, and decreases immune activity. Thus, glycolysis supports the growth and spread of tumors. All of this means that cancer cells are tied to their inefficient method of energy generation, so their need for glucose is very high.

This raises the question as to whether it is possible for us to lower our sugar consumption enough to deprive cancer cells of the fuel that they so desperately require. Research published in 2011 (Ho et al.) looked at whether a low-carbohydrate diet fed to mice could decrease blood sugar supply to cancer cells enough to slow their growth and even prevent new tumors from developing. The researchers fed mice two different diets: a low-carb, high-protein diet or a high-carb diet similar to the typical Western diet. The investigators were able to see that blood levels of glucose could be lowered from both an 8 percent carbohydrate diet (comparable to the amount of carbohydrate in the popular Atkins diet) as well as from a more sustainable 15 percent carbohydrate diet (with 58 percent protein and 26 percent fat). Both low-carb diets resulted in slower tumor growth than in the mice fed the Western diet.

Furthermore, adult mice that were genetically at a 70 percent to 80 percent lifetime risk for developing cancer were studied to see if a low-carb diet lowered their risk of cancer development. It was found that 30 percent of mice eating a low-carb diet developed cancer, whereas 70 percent of the mice on a normal typical Western type diet developed cancer. The researchers determined that the low-carbohydrate diets lowered insulin and therefore glucose uptake by cancer cells. Insulin is itself a growth factor for cancer cells, adding to this anticancer effect. While this study was done on mice and not humans, the results are thought-provoking. Low-carb diets lower blood sugar levels in humans. Thus, one could surmise that a low-carb diet may be an important dietary consideration to both prevent and impede cancer. Removing refined sugar and refined grains (think: pastries, pasta, white bread, and so on) are excellent strategies to lowering your carb intake and your blood glucose, and ultimately deterring potential cancer growth.

Cancer cells develop elaborate mechanisms to ensure they always have sufficient sugar supply. They even have increased insulin receptors on their surfaces so they can gobble up as much sugar as possible. When we consume a diet that consists primarily of simple carbohydrates and refined sugars, we are much more likely to develop insulin resistance. Insulin resistance is characterized by malfunctioning insulin receptors on our healthy cells and a compensatory increase in blood levels of insulin. Because cancer cells have so many insulin receptors, even in an insulin-resistant state, cancer cells will still have enough receptors to bind insulin. Over time, excessive refined sugar consumption can increase insulin levels and more selectively fuel cancer cells.

For all of these reasons, it is important to reduce or eliminate one's consumption of simple sugars (think: refined sugar, candy, most desserts, doughnuts). This does not mean that you should reduce the intake of foods with *naturally* occurring sugar, such as fruits and vegetables. The thousands of cancer-fighting compounds that fruits and vegetables contain far outweigh the potential harm from their sugar. We should focus on the types of sugar we consume, avoiding simple sugars rather than fruits and vegetables. If you have a stubborn sweet tooth, consider such sweeteners as stevia, date palm sugar, agave, honey, or maple syrup. Although these should be used with discretion, they are healthier options than artificial sweeteners.

Should I Avoid Chocolate?

Dark chocolate is a rich source of antioxidative and anti-inflammatory flavonoids. The flavonoids found in chocolate are similar to those found in green tea. The darker the chocolate—ideally at least 70 percent cocoa—the more flavonoids it contains. In fact, dark chocolate has twice the amount of flavonoids as does milk chocolate. Dark chocolate as a snack within a balanced diet has been demonstrated to improve DNA resistance to oxidative stress in humans for twenty-two hours, so daily consumption of dark chocolate provides the best continuous protection. If you limit your consumption to quantities of two ounces or less, the sugar in the chocolate is unlikely to cause blood sugar issues.

This is not true for prediabetics and diabetics, however, who should avoid chocolate sweetened with sugar. Organic dark chocolate that is minimally processed is the healthiest form of chocolate to eat. Remember, simple sugars other than those in dark chocolate should be avoided whenever possible.

Should I Avoid Bisphenol A (BPA)?

Bisphenol A is a type of toxin that can accumulate in our bodies. Sources of Bisphenol A include food and beverage containers, water bottles, plastic utensils, sales receipts printed on thermal paper, and baby bottles. The bad news is that we all should be very worried about BPA. Bisphenol A is toxic to our cells and is considered to be a cancer-causing chemical. The good news is that our bodies have a system—the detoxification pathway—in place to help us process those toxins. This system can get bogged down, but you can minimize your intake of BPA. The best way to reduce the amount of BPA in your diet is to reduce the amount of packaged and canned foods that you eat and drink.

A 2011 study (Betts) demonstrated that both BPA and bis (2-Ethylhexyl) phthalate (DEHP) were substantially reduced when the study participants stuck with a fresh foods diet versus foods that were canned and packed in plastic. This study actually showed a 66 percent reduction in BPA and upwards of a 56 percent reduction in DEHP in the urine of the study participants. Here are some other ways to reduce your exposure to toxins:

- Avoid using the microwave and *never* microwave food in plastic containers.
- Avoid drinking out of aluminum cans.
- Look at the number on the bottom of plastic bottles, inside the recycling symbol: numbers 2, 4, and 5 are okay; number 1 should be used only one time and then discarded; and numbers 3, 6, and 8 should be avoided entirely.
- Reduce your exposure to secondhand smoke, and if you smoke, quit.
- Eat organic.
- Decline sales receipts whenever possible.

In this modern age, it's impossible to avoid all toxins in our food and our environment. However, we can do things to reduce our exposure and support the body's internal detoxification pathway.

Should I Try a Vegetarian Diet?

The best cancer-prevention diet is a plant-based diet. Cancer prevention is associated with the consumption of five to ten servings of vegetables every day. This does not, however, mean that you can't eat meat. If you consume fish, free-range lean meats, and organically and grass-fed animals, you may obtain additional cancer-prevention benefits. If you prefer to eat a vegetarian diet, there can be many health benefits. Vegetarians report higher energy levels, fewer weight problems, and general enhanced well-being. A healthy vegetarian diet should include five to ten servings of vegetables a day and enough protein— typically 0.45 grams of protein per kilogram (2.2 pounds) of ideal body weight. That means that a 150-pound person should obtain a minimum of 30 grams of protein daily. If you are exercising daily, are pregnant, or have certain chronic diseases, your protein needs increase—often doubling or even tripling. Consuming sufficient protein while eating a vegetarian diet can be challenging and requires daily consumption of beans, legumes, tofu, nuts, and, in some cases, eggs.

Should I Try an Alkaline Diet?

There are a variety of diets purported to have cancer-prevention effects due to the alkaline nature of the foods they are based upon. Generally, alkaline diets emphasize fresh and raw vegetables, nuts, and citrus fruits, while avoiding refined sugar, meat, dairy, and alcohol. According to advocates of the alkaline diet, the typical modern Western diet produces residual acid, particularly phosphates, which are acidic, after metabolism. Vegetarian diets, which tend to be alkaline, cause a person to have more alkaline urine than do diets containing high amounts of meat and dairy products. The idea behind an alkaline diet is that it assists the body's effort to maintain its acid/alkaline balance by supplying alkaline buffers. The theory holds that without alkaline buffers, the body will ultimately pull alkaline minerals from the bone, causing decreased bone density. Although several clinical trials have failed to demonstrate such a bone demineralization effect, there may be some validity to the concept of an alkaline diet.

Proponents of the alkaline diet assert that the residual acidity of the typical Western diet leads to tissue degeneration and chronic inflammatory diseases. There is an association between acidosis and impaired immunity, reduced glutathione, and reduced insulin sensitivity. Even though the data supporting the benefits of reducing acidosis are still somewhat preliminary, the body of data is growing. Furthermore, if following an alkaline diet means there is an increased focus on fruits and vegetables and a reduction of processed foods, we are all for it. Alkaline diets do not need to be extreme to achieve health benefits. For most people, reducing acidosis is as simple as replacing table salt, sodium chloride, with potassium chloride and increasing daily consumption of fruits and vegetables. These changes can have significant positive benefits on cellular health and overall health.

Should I Try a Food Allergy Elimination Diet?

Food allergies are quite common, affecting as many as one in every three people. There is no proven link between consuming foods that create an immune-mediated allergic reaction (food allergens) and cancer. However, if an individual consumes food allergens repeatedly over months and years, there could be serious health consequences, including a predisposition to cancer development. Chronic consumption of food allergens impairs the health of all five of the body's key pathways (the immune system, inflammation, hormonal balance, insulin resistance, and digestion and detoxification). Food allergens can cause digestive distress that leads to a leaky gut and imbalanced bacteria in the intestinal tract. They can create chronic inflammation, which may manifest as joint pain, headaches, or sinusitis, among other ailments. Food allergies can contribute to insulin resistance and disrupt sugar balance. Allergen consumption favors humoral (antibody-driven) immunity over cytotoxic (direct cell-killing) immunity, which leads to autoimmune disease and impairs our cancer surveillance.

Eating food allergens disrupts the body's hormones, including perpetuating high levels of the stress hormone cortisol, which in turn suppresses immune function. So, although a direct link between consuming food allergens and cancer has not been established in the scientific literature, there are multiple indirect links that are concerning. Determining whether you have food allergies is best done under the guidance of a naturopathic doctor or integrative health care practitioner who can administer an allergy elimination and challenge diet and/or order a blood test, such as the lymphocyte response assay/ELISA ACT test. These tests identify immune reactivity to a panel of foods, helping to determine which foods may be allergens for you.

Should I Try a Wheat-Free Diet?

Wheat is an unusual grain. It is a hybridized grain that, on an evolutionary scale, is relatively new to our digestive tracts and immune systems. And we are a world addicted to wheat! Most of us consume wheat every day, often several times a day. Wheat is found in bread, many cereals, crackers, pastries, pasta, and cookies, and is even hidden in snack foods, soy sauce, and other foods. Wheat contains two proteins, gluten and gliadin, that can be quite problematic. In many individuals these proteins trigger an immune reaction in the digestive tract that is translated systemically. The systemic manifestation of this reaction can cause symptoms of chronic ill health (such as repeated headaches, joint pains, skin rashes, anxiety or depression, and abdominal pain or bloating) and can contribute to the development of such autoimmune diseases as multiple sclerosis, rheumatoid arthritis, and others.

There are some individuals who are especially sensitive to these wheat-based proteins, and if they continue to eat wheat, they will develop a serious inflammatory condition of their digestive tract called celiac disease. People with celiac disease need to avoid all gluten-containing foods. However, short of celiac disease, many more people have a milder form of wheat intolerance. Anyone who is struggling with persistent symptoms of ill health—stubborn weight gain, the inability to lose weight, unexplained fatigue, and especially digestive issues—may benefit from avoiding wheat.

The good news is that it is relatively easy to find out if you are likely to benefit from wheat avoidance. Avoiding wheat for three weeks will allow you to experience whether you feel better. If, after three weeks of avoidance, you are not sure, eat a good helping of wheat a few times a day for a couple of days, paying close attention to how you feel. This sudden reintroduction can unmask symptoms such as headaches, joint pains, insomnia, and so on that may have previously seemed just a part of your everyday life. If this wheat challenge produces symptoms, you would be best to avoid wheat. If you do this experiment, be sure to read labels because wheat is added to many foods that you wouldn't think of as wheat foods, such as some ketchups, tamari, beer, gravies, and salad dressings. Also, if you do determine that you need to avoid wheat, be sure to incorporate other fiber-rich foods into your daily diet to take the place of wheat.

Although there is no direct connection between wheat and cancer, any food that causes persistent ill health is putting stress on your body's five key pathways. The goal of living a cancer-preventive lifestyle is to minimize those habits and influences that impede health and, instead, to emphasize those things that support strong and consistent healthy internal pathways. This maximizes the quality of your life while removing strain and stress.

Should I Try a Detoxification Diet?

People often tell us with pride of the "brutal" detoxification or fasting type diet they undertake once or twice a year to totally cleanse their bodies. While these diets may have some benefit, they may also be jarring and inflammatory to the system. We believe in gentle detoxification throughout the year, which includes comprehensive support of the body's detoxification pathway. With its focus on whole foods, exercise, sleep, hydration, dietary supplements, and other aspects, our Five to Thrive diet and lifestyle plan does just that. If you would like a more intense detoxification experience, periodically remove all processed foods, sugar, and wheat from the diet, and eliminate alcohol and coffee altogether. Make sure you stay well hydrated to encourage daily bowel movements. Maintain this for three weeks for optimal benefit.

More comprehensive and sophisticated detoxification can be indicated for people with specific and known toxicities. Some people have high tissue levels of heavy metals or environmental chemicals that impair their health. These individuals will likely benefit from a tailored detoxification program developed by a naturopathic or integrative medical doctor with training in environmental medicine. It is important to undertake these types of detoxification programs under a doctor's guidance so that the impacts on the body and the effectiveness of the detox can be assessed. Please note that aggressive detoxification following cancer treatment should only be undertaken under the supervision of a qualified health care provider. There are websites listed in the Resource section that will help you find a health care professional in your area. Remember, ongoing detoxification can take place every moment of every day with the support of the Five to Thrive Plan.

Simple Steps to Create a Thriver's Diet

Changing how and what we eat is a lifelong project, and there is no better time to start than right now. Try to integrate a few of these simple ideas into your daily diet. You will feel better!

Add color to kill cancer. Choose fruits and vegetables from each of the color categories listed (see the table on page 70) and incorporate at least five different colors into your daily diet.

Know when to go organic. Yes, organic foods can be more expensive in some cases, but with certain foods it's absolutely critical. For example, thin-skinned fruits and berries should be organic as well as meat and dairy products. Check out the Environmental Working Group's website at www.ewg.org to find out which produce are the "dirtiest" and which foods are safe to be eaten in their nonorganic form.

Make eating an experience. Remember to slow down and truly enjoy the creation of food and the experience of nurturing yourself. As you eat, allow all of your senses to become engaged in the process.

Appreciate your food. Food has the power to harm and to heal. As you nourish and nurture yourself with food, admire and recognize its loving contribution to your health and your life.

CHAPTER 4

Core Strategy #4:

Utilize Dietary Supplements

We like to think of dietary supplements like prongs of a fork.
Precisely chiseled, these prongs are able to fit into the nooks and
crannies of our biochemical pathways to leverage their power.
Dietary supplements can create precise epigenetic changes in
the health of the five key pathways by influencing our internal
landscape on a cellular level. We receive many questions from
people regarding dietary supplement use. "There are so many
choices," they lament. "Where do I even begin?" While it's true
that countless dietary supplements could benefit our health and
have significant cancer-prevention actions, taking dozens of
supplements every day may not be feasible physically or finan-
cially. Dietary supplements are called "supplements" for a reason:
they are meant to supplement the diet and should not be used as
replacements for healthy eating. The role of dietary supplements
is to augment a healthy diet and lifestyle by providing additional,
targeted molecular support.

Following is an overview of what we consider to be the
five critical dietary supplements beneficial for *most* people. We
have selected the supplements that have the biggest potential to
improve health and help prevent cancer. This chapter will help

you prioritize which dietary supplements to take. The supplements we discuss are backed by scientific research and clinical experience. They were chosen because they influence all five key pathways of the body (the immune system, inflammation, hormonal balance, insulin resistance, and digestion and detoxification). Remember, when we effectively support the five pathways, we can change the epigenetic influences on our cells. Over time, this gentle yet precise impact can radically alter the terrain in your body and create an environment that impedes cancer development.

The Five Critical Action Steps

The five critical action steps in the dietary supplements strategy consist of using five groups of dietary supplements. These supplements have both short- and long-term benefits on our health as well as significant cancer-prevention actions. They are:

1. Omega-3 fatty acids

2. Probiotics

3. Polyphenols

4. Antioxidants

5. Vitamin D

Let's take a closer look at all five supplement groups, and how they connect to all five key pathways of the body.

Omega-3 Fatty Acids

Omega-3 fatty acids are part of a larger group of fats called essential fatty acids. In the body, omega-3 fatty acids are derived from alpha-linolenic acid (ALA). From ALA, the body makes all other omega-3 fatty acids, including eicosapentaenoic acid (EPA) and docosahexaenoic acid (DHA). Some individuals, however, cannot convert ALA into EPA or DHA because they lack sufficient activity of a critical enzyme needed for this conversion.

This metabolic challenge, combined with the fact that most people don't ingest large enough quantities of ALA, has led to a populationwide deficiency in omega-3 fatty acids. That's why omega-3 is a foundation in the Five to Thrive dietary supplement strategy.

Omega-3 fatty acids are naturally found in fish, fish oils, vegetables, nuts, and seeds. The only vegetable oils that contain EPA and DHA are those from sea vegetables (such as kelp, dulce, and nori); land-based plants only contain the precursor, ALA. Nonhydrogenated canola oil, flaxseed, walnuts, and other nuts and seeds are particularly rich sources of ALA. The typical North American diet includes about 1 to 3 grams of ALA each day. However, the typical North American diet lacks EPA and DHA, providing only 0.10 to 0.15 grams per day. This diet contains high amounts—as much as 12 to 15 grams—of omega-6 fatty acids such as linoleic acid. That means that most people have an overabundance of omega-6, with deficiencies in omega-3 fatty acids—particularly EPA and DHA. A high ratio of omega-6 to omega-3 fatty acids is as dangerous as an overt deficiency of the omega-3 fatty acids. This imbalanced ratio predisposes the body to inflammation, alters immune function, increases insulin resistance, and increases cellular susceptibility to damage. As you might suspect, omega-3 fatty acids positively influence all five key pathways of the body (see chart, opposite)!

Cancer-Prevention Effects: Omega-3 Fatty Acids

Ingestion of omega-3 fatty acids has been linked with decreased risk for a variety of cancers in clinical trials. People at high risk for colon cancer treated with omega-3 fatty acids for thirty days had decreased tumor cell proliferation as well as decreased inflammatory activity. Women with the highest intake of marine-derived omega-3 fatty acids lowered their risk of developing adenomatous polyps of the colon (precancerous growths) by 33 percent, compared to the lowest intake group. In a 2010 study (West et al.), adults with a history of familial polyposis who took

The Positive Influence of Omega-3 Fatty Acids

KEY PATHWAY	BENEFITS
The Immune System	• Improve overall immune function: Intake of EPA and DHA lowers the omega-6 to omega-3 ratio, which is correlated with enhanced immunity and reduced infections. • Activate immune cells: Supplementation with low dosages of DHA improves lymphocyte activation.
Inflammation	• Change cell signaling: Omega-3 fatty acids influence cellular membranes and change critical cell-signaling mechanisms, in turn, altering gene expression. • Reduce inflammatory biomarkers: Intake of EPA and DHA reduces many of the inflammatory molecules (such as C-reactive protein, interleukin-6, and homocysteine) that tend to be elevated in people with aggressive cancers. In people with colon cancer receiving chemotherapy, supplemented fish oil reduced C-reactive protein.
Hormonal Balance	• Reduce stress-induced cortisol elevation: Supplementing with EPA has been found to improve depression, an effect linked to its ability to reduce cortisol. • Modulate hormonal activity in ER+ cancer cells: Supplementation inhibits estrogen receptor–driven cell growth pathways in ER+ breast cancer cells.
Insulin Resistance	• Increase insulin sensitivity: Even in obese, insulin-resistant adults, a diet high in cod increases insulin sensitivity. • Reduce triglycerides: A 2012 meta-analysis (Lopez-Huertas) showed that supplementation with at least 1 gram per day of omega-3 fatty acid for at least three months significantly reduces triglycerides, a marker of insulin resistance and metabolic syndrome, by up to 25 percent.
Digestion and Detoxification	• Upregulate detoxification genes: Consumption of EPA and DHA upregulates Nrf2-regulated gene expression. Nrf2 gene codes for various detoxification proteins. • Support intestinal repair: Long-chain fatty acids such as EPA and DHA are particularly effective in supporting intestinal barrier integrity by improving resistance to damaging agents and reducing inflammation-mediated permeability.

2 grams of EPA daily lowered their risk of developing colonic polyps by 22 percent compared with those who took a placebo. Supplemental omega-3 fatty acids have also been shown to reduce the pro-inflammatory and immunosuppressive reaction to ultraviolet radiation in human skin, thereby reducing risk for nonmelanoma skin cancer.

Omega-3 fatty acids from flaxseed have been demonstrated to inhibit breast cancer cell growth and exert antiestrogen effects. This seems to be the result of both the essential fatty acids and the other compounds in flaxseed known as lignans. There is also evidence that omega-3 ingestion can help prevent prostate cancer growth because of its anti-inflammatory effects; however, the scientific evidence for omega-3s and prostate cancer prevention is mixed. Researchers from New Zealand (Norrish et al.) found that men with the highest consumption of fish and associated highest blood levels of EPA and DHA had a 40 percent reduced risk of prostate cancer.

In patients diagnosed with lung cancer, supplementation with EPA and DHA concurrent with chemotherapy reduced blood markers of inflammation, which lowered the risk for cachexia (severe malnutrition). EPA and DHA supplementation also increases the efficacy of chemotherapy given to people with advanced non-small-cell lung cancer, laying the groundwork for increased survival.

Finding the Best Supplement: Omega-3 Fatty Acids

It can be difficult to consume enough omega-3 fatty acids every day to get the anticancer benefits, but a variety of EPA and DHA supplements are available. The most important factor when choosing an EPA and DHA supplement is to evaluate the quality of the supplement, particularly for those oils extracted from fish. Many forms of marine life are now contaminated with high levels of heavy metals (such as mercury) and other pollutants that are independently linked with cancer risk, and these can show up in supplements. The extraction process of EPA and DHA can be done with a bleaching process that uses dioxin, a cancer-causing substance. If this dioxin is not removed from the final product, it will be present in the fish oil supplements.

Another important parameter of fish oil quality involves freshness. Fish oil that has been poorly extracted can become rancid. These products tend to have a strong fishy odor, and their health benefits are questionable. When purchasing an EPA and DHA supplement, look for a third-party certification quality seal on the label. It is worth the time to contact the manufacturer and ask them about their manufacturing process and ask for a copy of their certificate of analysis for the lot of product that you have purchased. This certificate of analysis should demonstrate that the product has been tested for, and is absent of, heavy metals, dioxins, and rancidity. Some companies post these certificates of analyses on their websites. Integrative health care practitioners can also guide you to the best quality fish oil supplements.

Dosage of essential fatty acids varies, but as a general rule two capsules daily is a standard dose. Omega-3 fatty acids from fish oil should be standardized to contain EPA and DHA, usually in the vicinity of 300 milligrams EPA and 200 milligrams DHA per 1,000 milligram capsule of fish oil. Omega-3 fatty acids from flax oil (one tablespoon daily) are usually made from cold-pressed seed oil and contain approximately 60 percent omega-3 fatty acids. Supplemental omega-3 oils are best tolerated when taken with food to avoid nausea and an unpleasant burping of fish oil. If you're having trouble with the odor, try freezing the capsules and taking them frozen. Individuals on Coumadin (a blood-thinning medication) should alert their health care practitioners about their fish oil or flaxseed oil supplementation as it may affect their INR (International Normalized Ratio) test results, which is the standard test used to measure blood "stickiness" in people taking Coumadin. Individuals with fish allergies should not take fish oil capsules but may benefit from plant-based omega-3 products, such as algae-based oil or flaxseed oil.

Probiotics

Who would think that using bacteria would be one of the foundational cancer-prevention action steps in the Five to Thrive Plan? Beneficial bacteria, also known as commensal bacteria or probiotics, are in fact essential ingredients in our supplement strategy. We rely on these beneficial bacteria for a variety of vital functions. The bacteria in the intestinal tract help metabolize vitamins into their absorbable and bioactive components, bind waste products for removal in stool, and help regulate immunity.

Our bodies are colonized with bacteria during birth and with early breastfeeding. Afterward, we maintain bacteria through the foods we eat—particularly fermented foods such as miso, yogurt, fresh sauerkraut, and kefir. Because our bodies cannot produce bacteria, we rely upon external sources (food and supplements) to replenish and maintain the bacteria that we have. Unfortunately, daily living can take its toll on the quantity and type of bacteria in our bodies. One of the ways we destroy our beneficial bacterial population is through the use of antibiotics. Although antibiotics can be immensely helpful and even life-saving, they are indiscriminate and kill many of the body's helpful bacteria while they're killing the bad bacteria. Unless we replace these beneficial bacteria after taking antibiotics, the digestive tract becomes imbalanced and overridden with harmful bacteria, creating a condition called dysbiosis. People with a dysbiotic bowel lack beneficial bacteria and tend to have an overgrowth of disease-causing bacteria.

Dysbiosis also leads to leaky gut syndrome. "Leaky gut" is a term used to describe when the intestinal lining becomes weak and permeable, allowing food particles, antigens, and toxins to enter the system. Unfortunately, as we age, intestinal resilience decreases, and we are more susceptible to dysbiosis, intestinal inflammation, and leaky gut. The connection between dysbiosis and overall health is a significant and far-reaching one. From a cancer–prevention perspective, dysbiosis significantly impacts each of the body's five key pathways.

The Positive Influence of Probiotics

KEY PATHWAY	BENEFITS
The Immune System	• Improve the immune response: A 2012 randomized placebo controlled trial (Reale et al.) was conducted on seventy-two healthy Italian blue-collar male smokers randomly divided for daily intake of *Lactobacillus casei* powder or placebo. Cigarette smoking reduces natural killer (NK) activity, and three weeks of supplementation with the *Lactobacillus* prevented the smoke-dependent expected NK activity reduction, and in fact, improved cytotoxic immunity. • Increase resistance to infection: In a 2005 study (de Vrese et al.) adults who received oral probiotics had significantly decreased cold symptoms as well as shorter duration of common cold episodes.
Inflammation	• Decrease inflammatory cytokines: A 2010 pilot study of elderly persons (Mikelsaar et al.) found that the intestinal load of lactobacilli was linked to markers of inflammation, including elevated white blood cells, lowered blood glucose, and decreased content of oxidized low-density lipoprotein. • Reduce systemic inflammatory diseases: Improvement of atopic eczema/dermatitis and food allergy have been demonstrated with the use of *Lactobacillus rhamnosus* GG, which alleviates intestinal inflammation.
Hormonal Balance	• Reduce depression and anxiety: A randomized controlled trial (Messaoudi et al.) of fifty-five healthy people who received either thirty days of a probiotic supplement (*Lactobacillus helveticus* and *Bifidobacterium longum*) or placebo (inactive substance) found that those taking the probiotic had reduced depression, irritability, and anxiety and increased coping ability in response to stress.

The Positive Influence of Probiotics, *continued*

KEY PATHWAY   BENEFITS

Insulin
Resistance
- Improve insulin sensitivity: Probiotics, particularly *Lactobacillus* spp. and *Bifidobacterium* spp., improve glucose tolerance, lower insulin levels, and maintain insulin sensitivity. In a 2010 randomized trial (Andreasen et al.), forty-five males with type 2 diabetes, impaired, or normal glucose tolerance who received *Lactobacillus acidophilus* NCFM experienced improved insulin sensitivity, whereas it worsened in the placebo group.

Digestion and
Detoxification
- Improve intestinal integrity: Probiotics preserve intestinal integrity and maintain a healthy intestinal barrier. This effect has been shown to reduce intestinal bloating in functional digestive disturbances such as irritable bowel syndrome. A 2012 randomized trial (Z.H. Liu et al.) demonstrated that probiotic treatment can reduce the rate of postoperative infection and is associated with reduced markers of intestinal permeability.
- Prevent intestinal infections: Lactobacilli reduce the severity of intestinal infections with *H. pylori* and various fungal organisms as well as decrease the rate of infectious complications in patients undergoing colectomy for colorectal cancer.
- Minimize liver inflammation: People with dysbiosis are at increased risk for developing elevations of the inflammatory marker TNF-alpha and ultimately liver inflammation. A 2010 study (Rifatbegovic et al.) assessed 120 patients who underwent liver resection due to hepatitis C and cirrhosis; those who received probiotics for three days prior to and for seven days after surgery experienced faster recovery, better acute immune responses, fewer postsurgical complications, and lower mortality rates than those who were not using probiotics.

Cancer-Prevention Effects: Probiotics

Given its direct support of each of the body's five key pathways, probiotic use has been linked directly to cancer prevention. One clinical trial (Rafter et al.) randomized 398 Japanese adults with a previous history of colon cancer to receive either dietary fiber from wheat bran or *Lactobacillus casei*, a probiotic. After four years they were examined by colonoscopy for new tumors. Among the subjects taking the wheat bran, the risk of developing new tumors was unaffected. However, in the subjects taking *Lactobacillus*, the chance of developing a colon cancer recurrence was reduced by 24 percent. Although the trial was small, similar results have been demonstrated in several other clinical trials. A literature review published in 2008 (Fotiadis et al.) concluded that probiotics, prebiotics, and synbiotics (a probiotic plus a type of fiber that supports the growth of the probiotic) have great potential for both the prevention and the treatment of colon cancer. After twelve weeks of supplementation, the synbiotic group demonstrated improvements in several colon cancer biomarkers. The intervention significantly reduced the rate of colon cell proliferation, improved gut integrity, and decreased exposure of colon cells to cancer-causing chemicals. Synbiotic consumption also altered the cytokine secretion pattern, leading to increased immunity.

Other research suggests a protective role of probiotics on the stomach, potentially lowering the risk of stomach cancer. Some preclinical research studies suggest probiotics might reduce the risk of liver and bladder cancer. Several mechanisms could explain the preventive action of probiotics against cancer, including alteration of the intestinal microflora; inactivation of cancer-causing compounds; improvement of immune response; antiproliferative effects; fermentation of undigested food; and inhibition of cell-signaling growth pathways.

Finding the Best Supplement: Probiotics

Probiotics can be taken as single strains of *Lactobacillus* or *Bifidobacterium* or as combinations of several different bacterial species. All of these supplements have the potential to be beneficial. The single-species probiotics work because *Lactobacillus* spp. and *Bifidobacterium* spp. are the most common and dominant bacteria in our intestines. These bacteria survive well in there, and when present in sufficient quantities, they create an intestinal pH that facilitates colonization by other beneficial bacterial. Combination probiotics supply a variety of the beneficial bacteria, which may facilitate the reestablishment of a healthy balance of bacteria in the bowel more quickly. Some probiotic supplements also contain prebiotics, compounds that feed and protect the beneficial bacteria. These can include things like lactoferrin, fructooligosaccharide (FOS), and a beneficial yeast known as *Saccharomyces boulardii*. This combination of probiotic (bacteria) and prebiotic are often called synbiotics and are particularly indicated for long-term use because the prebiotic actually enhances the viability of the probiotic.

The most common quality issue related to probiotics is inadequate potency. Probiotics are living organisms, which means they eventually die. High-quality probiotic products have strategies in place to reduce the die-off of these bacteria. These include the use of high-quality probiotics packaged in blister packs or dark glass bottles. Other quality issues include inappropriate identification of the bacterial species or strain and use of a strain that has not been shown to be effective in humans. When purchasing a probiotic, it is important to make sure there is research documenting the strain's use in humans. Consulting with a qualified integrative health care practitioner or pharmacist will provide you with guidance to obtain the best product. There is no recommended daily allowance for probiotics, and dosing can vary significantly depending on the user's age, medical conditions, and medications as well as quality of the product. Generally speaking, probiotic supplementation is recommended between 10 million and 10 billion colony-forming units (CFU) daily.

To prevent dysbiosis from antibiotic use, we recommend probiotics be taken concurrently with antibiotics and for several weeks after the course of antibiotics has ended. But then again, if you are following this plan, you are already taking probiotics on a daily basis and will continue to do so even if you are prescribed an antibiotic. It is best to take the probiotic at a different time of day than the antibiotic. Probiotics are very safe, except in people who have a significantly decreased white blood cell count (below normal). In this instance, probiotics should not be taken because of the reported risk of septicemia (blood infection).

Polyphenols

Polyphenols are one of the main reasons we advocate a colorful diet full of vegetables and fruits. One of the most healthful types of polyphenols are the thousands of colorful flavonoids present in foods; however, there are a few that stand out for their cancer-prevention actions. From a dietary supplement standpoint, we have three favorite flavonoids:

1. Green tea flavonoid catechins and L-theanine

2. Curcumin from turmeric root

3. Resveratrol from red grape skins, peanuts, and small berries

There are many other exciting flavonoids to keep an eye on. Some of the more scientifically interesting polyphenols are cocoa from chocolate, ellagic acid and anthocyanins from berries and pomegranates, delphinidin from berries—especially the maca berry—and quercetin from apples and onions. As more human clinical trials examine the effects of these compounds, we expect to see some exciting new prevention options revealed. Let's take a closer look at the unique cancer-prevention profile of green tea, turmeric, and grape-skin flavonoids.

Green Tea (Epigallocatechin Gallate and L-theanine)

Green tea is processed from the leaves of the tea plant, *Camellia sinensis*. Although all forms of traditional tea come from this plant, green tea is processed differently from black and oolong teas. For green tea, immediately after the tea leaves are picked, they are steamed to stop the fermentation process and then dried. Black tea is fermented fully by drying the leaves for many hours, rolling them to release additional enzymes, and drying further. Oolong tea is a partially fermented tea. By minimizing the fermentation process in green tea, more of the naturally present chemicals found in tea are preserved. Green tea is rich in catechins (polyphenols), vitamins, minerals, and amino acids (such as L-theanine). It also has caffeine, but only about two-thirds of the amount as coffee. Caffeine content increases with additional fermentation, so black tea has more caffeine than green tea does.

Of the catechins in green tea, epigallocatechin gallate (EGCG) is the most well-studied compound. Another important constituent in green tea is L-theanine, an amino acid. Green tea has been studied in humans for prevention of heart disease, obesity, and cancer. The potential benefit in these conditions is the result of green tea's effect on each of the body's five key pathways. Remember, this is how we prioritize the herbs and nutrients that make it to the foundation plan—by how many of the pathways they positively influence. Green tea touches all five (see chart, opposite)!

Cancer-Prevention Effects. The evidence supporting green tea's cancer-prevention effects comes from large and small population studies. While these types of studies are not as definitive as double-blinded clinical trials, they are very helpful in assessing the long-term impact of green tea as a part of day-to-day life, which is exactly how prevention works. A good portion of the research on green tea has been done on *drinking* green tea as opposed to *taking* green tea supplements. Keep in mind that when research mentions one cup, it means a traditional Japanese

The Positive Influence of Green Tea

KEY PATHWAY	BENEFITS
The Immune System	• Stimulates T cells: L-theanine is broken down into ethylamine, which specifically activates T lymphocytes to proliferate and secrete interferon gamma, increasing immune reactivity against viruses and cancer. • Antimicrobial: EGCG can kill bacteria and viruses, including the influenza virus.
Inflammation	• Antioxidant: Green tea flavonoids exert antioxidant effects, decreasing the formation of lipid peroxides (oxidants). • Anti-inflammatory: Epigallocatechin gallate (EGCG) inhibits the initial inflammatory response to ultraviolet-B (UVB) radiation, thereby reducing cellular damage. • Inhibits tissue inflammation: EGCG inhibits matrix metalloproteinases, which are released in inflamed tissue and allow inflammation to spread.
Hormonal Balance	• Reduces the stress response: L-theanine increases dopamine and serotonin production and generates alpha waves in the central nervous system, resulting in lower blood pressure and reduced anxiety (causing a relaxed yet alert state). • Modulates hormonal activity in fat cells: Inhibits fat cell proliferation and differentiation and may decrease release of obesity-related hormones.
Insulin Resistance	• Stimulates fat oxidation: EGCG stimulates fat metabolism into energy and has been shown in some clinical trials to support healthy weight. • Inhibits IGF-1: EGCG has been shown to inhibit insulin growth factor-1 activation, which, like insulin, stimulates the growth of cancer cells.
Digestion and Detoxification	• Decreases activation of carcinogens: In vitro studies show that EGCG stimulates cytochrome P450 detoxification enzymes and blocks the mutagenic (DNA-damaging) effects of carcinogens.

cup (about 100 milliliters or 3.5 ounces). A typical American mug of tea is about 8 ounces.

Prostate cancer is perfectly suited to the prevention benefits of green tea because this form of cancer typically takes decades to grow, giving ample opportunity to use targeted cancer-prevention strategies like green tea over a long period of time. In a 2006 study (Bettuzzi et al.), sixty volunteers with high-grade prostate intraepithelial neoplasia, a precancerous condition, participated in a double-blind, placebo-controlled study. The treatment group took green tea capsules, totaling 600 milligrams every day. After one year, only one tumor was diagnosed among the thirty men taking the green tea capsules, whereas nine cancers were found among the thirty placebo-treated men. Total prostate-specific antigen (PSA) was lower in the green tea group than in the placebo-treated men. Assuming this effect continues year after year, this indicates strong cancer-prevention potential for green tea extract.

Cancers of the digestive tract also seem to respond to the preventive effects of green tea. In one study (Z. Chen et al.) there was a protective effect from drinking low-temperature green tea. Specifically, there was a 31 percent decrease in the risk of developing esophageal cancer. Of note, hot-temperature tea increases the risk, with the damage from the high temperature outweighing the benefit of the green tea. Another study (Setiawan et al.) found that green tea drinking reduced the incidence of chronic gastritis, or inflammation and ulceration of the stomach, which is a risk factor for stomach cancer.

A double-blind, randomized trial published in 2008 (Shimizu et al.) studied 136 adults with a history of colon polyps (a cancer risk factor) and assessed the impact of green tea on the development of colon cancer. The treatment group took 1,500 milligrams of green tea extract tablets that were standardized to 80 percent catechins and also drank six (3.5-ounce) cups of green tea daily for one year. The control group only drank the green tea. After a year, all participants underwent a colonoscopy.

The results were that 31 percent of those who did not take the tablets developed at least one colon polyp, whereas only 15 percent of the treatment group developed one or more polyp. The addition of the green tea supplement lowered the risk of colon polyps by 50 percent. This is an important study because it shows that quantity matters. By adding the capsules, the daily consumption of green tea was raised to more than ten cups daily—a quantity that is most consistently associated with cancer prevention across all cancer types. This study also indicates the role supplements can play in boosting the level of green tea—great news for people who can't drink ten cups of green tea every day. Plus, green tea capsules are over 99 percent caffeine-free.

Green tea extract may be particularly effective for the blood-borne cancer known as chronic lymphocytic leukemia. In a 2013 phase 2 study (Shanafelt et al.) forty-two previously untreated patients with Rai stage 0 to II chronic lymphocytic leukemia were given a standardized extract of green tea, Polyphenon E, at 2,000 milligrams twice daily for up to six months. At the conclusion of the study, 31 percent of patients experienced a sustained reduction of greater than twenty in their white blood cell counts, and 69 percent of patients with palpable lymph nodes experienced at least a 50 percent reduction in the sum of all involved nodes. The green tea was also well tolerated.

Breast cancer has also been shown in population studies to respond positively to green tea. A study in 2001 (Inoue et al.) of 1,160 postsurgical women with breast cancer demonstrated that those who drank three or more cups of green tea daily (average consumption was five cups daily) had a 31 percent decreased risk of breast cancer recurrence over their non–tea drinking counterparts. For the women with early (stages I and II) breast cancer, the protective effects of green tea equaled a 51 percent reduction in recurrence. A similar effect was found in a 1998 study (Nakachi et al.), which studied 472 Japanese women diagnosed with breast cancer. Women with early stage breast cancer who drank at least five cups of green tea (average of seven cups) daily had an

8 percent reduction in recurrence rate, and the recurrences were delayed by almost a full year compared with women who drank fewer than four cups of green tea daily (average was two cups).

One 2010 study (Iwasaki et al.) questions the breast cancer-preventive actions of green tea. This large study featured more than fifty-three thousand Japanese women living in Japan and followed them for an average of 13.6 years. The participants' green tea drinking was reported in a questionnaire at the beginning of the study and then again every five years. The researchers concluded that the amount of green tea consumed had no impact on the risk of breast cancer. Although the results of this study are at odds with previous research, there may be some explanations. The women in this study had a very low incidence of breast cancer, and it may be that in a population of women already at relatively low risk, frequent green tea consumption is not an impactful prevention strategy. This means that women at higher risk of breast cancer (like the women with a previous diagnosis of breast cancer in the earlier studies) are the ones most likely to benefit from green tea's preventive actions. The lack of benefit in this study may also be because the typical Japanese diet is already very high in a variety of flavonoids from soy and vegetables. Adding more flavonoids such as those found in green tea may not add more benefit to a diet already rich in protection. If this is true, women eating six to eight servings of vegetables and fruits daily may not get the protective benefits from green tea, but women eating fewer servings may benefit greatly from it.

Several large population studies (Liu, Xing, and Fei; Yuan, Sun, and Butler) have demonstrated the protective benefits of green tea against the development of cancers of the cervix, lung, bladder, and head and neck. Green tea supports detoxification, provides antioxidant protection, and helps create a state of relaxed alertness.

Finding the Best Supplement. A variety of green tea supplements are available. Many contain the ingredient Sunphenon, which we recommend because it is properly standardized and is made of highly purified organic polyphenols found naturally in green tea. A 300 milligram capsule of green tea extract that is standardized to contain at least 50 percent catechins, preferably 80 percent catechins, of which at least 45 percent is EGCG, is equivalent to two Japanese cups of tea. The Sunphenon ingredient contains greater than 80 percent polyphenols and catechins. To achieve the equivalent of ten cups daily (assuming that you are not also *drinking* green tea), you would need to take four to five capsules daily. To take and drink green tea safely, always take it with food.

For antianxiety, blood pressure–lowering, and additional antioxidant affects, look for an extract standardized to contain L-theanine (brand name Suntheanine) at 100 milligrams per capsule. The typical dose of L-theanine is 200 to 300 milligrams. Green tea extracts should be chosen with care. Commercially grown green tea contains pesticide residue, which can remain in the green tea extract. Green tea extract may also contain carcinogenic solvent residues. It is important to learn from the manufacturer how they ensure that each batch of their green tea extracts are solvent-free and pesticide-free. Generally, the best-quality green tea is made from organically grown plants, and each batch is screened for solvent residues. Quality green tea extract is generally considered quite safe. However, it can alter the effectiveness of other medications such as Coumadin, oral contraceptives, and beta-blockers. In some people, high doses of green tea can cause anxiety, tremors, palpitations, and insomnia. Green tea can also cause weight loss, which can actually be an added benefit for some people.

Curcumin

Curcumin refers to a large group of flavonoids known as curcuminoids found in the root of the turmeric plant (*Curcuma longa*). Turmeric is part of the traditional diets in many Asian countries. It has been used in Asian and Ayurvedic systems of medicine for centuries as an anti-inflammatory, digestive aid, and liver tonic.

Curcumin has been researched extensively around the world. One of the challenges with curcumin is that it is poorly absorbed from the digestive tract into the blood. As little as 15 percent (perhaps up to 60 percent) of orally consumed curcumin is absorbed intact.

Because of the poor absorption profile and rapid absorption of curcumin, relatively few clinical studies have been conducted to determine if the wide range of physiological activities of curcumin are applicable in humans. However, the metabolic products of curcumin, particularly demethoxycurcumin and bisdemethoxycurcumin, are absorbed more readily and appear to be biologically active. Specialized preparations of curcumin can enhance its absorption and bioavailability.

The Positive Influence of Curcumin

KEY PATHWAY	BENEFITS
The Immune System	• Reduces T cell–induced inflammation: Curcumin inhibits T cell NF-kB activation (this comes from an animal study).
	• Antimicrobial: Turmeric extract and the essential oil of *Curcuma longa* inhibit the growth of a variety of bacteria, parasites, and pathogenic fungi.
Inflammation	• Antioxidant: In vitro studies have shown that curcuminoids exert potent antioxidant effects and enhance cellular resistance to oxidative damage.
	• Anti-inflammatory: Curcuminoids exert liver-protective effects, in part because of reduced production of inflammatory cytokines.
	• Inhibits NF-kB: Curcumin potently downregulates NF-kB and in so doing inhibits the amplification of the inflammatory response.
Hormonal Balance	• Increases resistance to stress: Curcumin is effective in alleviating chronic stress-induced disorders in rodents by modulating neuroendocrine functions of the central nervous system.
	• Modifies cortisol secretion: Curcumin inhibits cortisol secretion stimulated by adrenal corticotropin hormone (ACTH), which helps reestablish the sensitivity of the stress-response axis.

KEY PATHWAY	BENEFITS
Insulin Resistance	• Reduces insulin resistance: In vitro and animal studies have shown that curcumin downregulates the inflammatory cytokines resistin and leptin, upregulates adiponectin, and alters signal transduction pathways. The net effect of these actions is a reversal of insulin resistance, high blood sugar, elevated lipids, and other inflammatory symptoms associated with obesity and metabolic diseases.
Digestion and Detoxification	• Improves digestion: Curcumin inhibits intestinal spasm and increases digestive enzyme secretion (as shown in animal studies). • Protects against ulcer formation: Turmeric has been shown in animals to inhibit ulcer formation caused by stress, alcohol, and medications. This effect has been demonstrated in a clinical trial of twenty-five patients with endoscopically diagnosed gastric ulcer. Taking 600 milligrams of powdered turmeric five times daily resulted in complete healing of the ulcers after twelve weeks of treatment. • Supports detoxification: Curcumin exerts potent antioxidant effects in the liver, protecting liver cells from oxidative stress, and increases bile output and solubility, which supports the elimination of fat-soluble toxins.

Cancer-Prevention Effects. In vitro (test tube) and animal studies have shown that curcumin inhibits cancer formation at all stages of development; it protects cells against initial damage from cancer-causing compounds, slows tumor growth, stimulates apoptosis of cancer cells, and prevents the formation of blood vessels necessary for tumor growth. Curcumin has been shown to inhibit the growth of colon, breast, prostate, and melanoma cancer cell lines.

Curcumin has also been studied clinically in humans. Curcumin extract has been shown in clinical trials to inhibit the growth of colon and pancreatic cancers. The trials are small and preliminary, and the impact of curcumin from a prevention standpoint is not well understood. However, given the pronounced anticancer effect of curcumin seen in in vitro and animal studies from the vast number of genes and pathways that curcumin modifies, the prevention potential for curcumin is significant. A 2006 study (Cruz-Correa et al.) demonstrating this potential was done on people with familial adenomatous polyposis (FAP), which is a risk factor for colon cancer. In this study, five patients with FAP received 480 milligrams of curcumin and 20 milligrams of quercetin (another plant-derived flavonoid) orally three times daily for six months before colon removal. The number of polyps decreased by 60 percent, and the size of polyps decreased by 50 percent in the removed colons. These patients tolerated the treatment well and without side effects.

Another study published in 2001 (Cheng et al.) found that of twenty-five individuals at high risk of cancer who had premalignant lesions, curcumin intake was associated with decreased progression of cancer in 50 percent of patients with recently surgically removed bladder cancer, 28 percent of patients with oral leukoplakia (a precancerous condition of the mouth), 16 percent of patients with intestinal metaplasia of the stomach (a precancerous condition of the stomach), and 25 percent of patients with cervical intraepithelial neoplasm (a precancerous condition of the cervix). Another form of cancer, multiple myeloma, may be deterred with curcumin. A 2012 trial (Golombick et al.) studied thirty-six patients with two precancerous conditions that can progress to multiple myeloma. The trial found that both 4 gram and 8 gram daily doses of curcumin reduced progression to multiple myeloma, whereas a placebo had no effect.

Although more clinical trials are needed to further determine the direct potential of curcumin specific to cancer prevention, because it positively influences all five of the body's key pathways, it is a foundational supplement in the Five to Thrive Plan.

Finding the Best Supplement. One of the challenges with curcumin supplementation is finding a form that is absorbable and bioavailable. We recommend supplements that contain the curcumin extracts Theracurmin, Mervia, or BCM-95 for superior absorption and bioavailability. Please note that we do not recommend the long-term use of curcumin supplements with piperine, which is added to increase absorption, because piperine interacts with a wide spectrum of prescription medications; it also increases the absorption of other toxins from the digestive tract. Any form of curcumin should be tested to be free of solvent residues, pesticides, and heavy metals. These tests should be made available to you upon request for the lot of any curcumin product that you purchase.

The dosage of curcumin for cancer prevention is largely unknown. The few prevention studies that have been done have demonstrated benefit with ranges of 480 milligrams to 2,000 milligrams of curcumin. Studies of patients with active cancers have demonstrated benefit from curcumin at higher doses, typically in the range of 4,000 milligrams to 8,000 milligrams of a simple curcumin extract. The use of curcumin extracts significantly increases the bioavailabity of curcumin, allowing for lower effective doses. Depending on the extract, it could be from 600 milligrams to 2,000 milligrams daily. Curcumin is well tolerated, other than causing occasional mild digestive upset. Curcumin inhibits certain cytochrome P450 detoxification enzymes (CYP1A2) and enhances others (CYP2A6), so it may interfere with other medications. If you are taking medications, it is important to consult with a qualified integrative health care practitioner or a pharmacist before starting curcumin.

Resveratrol

Resveratrol is a naturally occurring polyphenol found in red grapes, peanuts, and some berries. These plants produce resveratrol in response to stress, fungal infection, and injury. This means that the amount of resveratrol can vary from, for instance, one grape vine to another depending on the stresses that each vine is exposed to. Resveratrol has three forms: a trans- and a cis form

The Positive Influence of Resveratrol

KEY PATHWAY	BENEFITS
The Immune System	• Reduces autoimmunity: In vitro studies have demonstrated that resveratrol supports immune tolerance and may reduce autoimmune reactivity. • Lowers inflammatory immune reactions: In vitro studies have shown that resveratrol reduces T lymphocyte overactivation and therefore pro-inflammatory cytokines.
Inflammation	• Antioxidant: In vitro studies have shown that resveratrol exerts antioxidant effects by neutralizing pro-oxidants. • Anti-inflammatory: In vitro studies demonstrate anti-inflammatory actions of resveratrol by inhibiting inflammatory cyclooxygenase (COX) and lipoxygenase (LOX) enzymes as well as NF kappa B and TNF alpha. This is the result of resveratrol modifying the expression of many inflammatory genes.
Hormonal Balance	• Modulates estrogen receptors: In vitro studies have shown that resveratrol stimulates estrogen receptors, particularly when there is a low level of estrogen present. In the presence of estrogen, resveratrol blocks the action of the estrogen receptor in vitro.
Insulin Resistance	• Lowers IGF-1: Resveratrol downregulates insulin-like growth factor-1 (IGF-1). IGF-1 is a growth factor for many cancers. A 2010 clinical study (Brown et al.) found that ingestion of 2.5 grams of resveratrol significantly reduced IGF-1 in forty subjects after one month of consumption.
Digestion and Detoxification	• Decreases activation of carcinogens: In vitro studies show that resveratrol inhibits certain cytochrome P450 detoxification enzymes. This could reduce the activation of some carcinogens. • Increases detoxification: In vitro studies show that resveratrol increases the binding, or conjugating enzymes, used in the second phase of detoxification, promoting the elimination of cancer-causing compounds.

and a methylated form called pterostilbene. Trans-resveratrol is the most studied form in animals and humans. Pterostilbene is mostly produced rather than extracted and is also the subject of an increasing number of studies. The majority of research on resveratrol is preclinical research done on cells or in animals. This research has demonstrated impressive anticancer potential that has fueled significant interest in resveratrol.

Cancer-Prevention Effects. One question that has plagued researchers is whether resveratrol is even absorbed when taken orally. In an effort to determine this, a small clinical trial (Patel et al.) of twenty people with colon cancer consumed eight daily doses of resveratrol at 500 milligrams or 1 gram before surgical removal of their colon tumors. Resveratrol was found to be well tolerated. Tissue samples found both resveratrol and its metabolites in the removed colon tissue and cancer cells, indicating that it was absorbed. Consumption of resveratrol reduced the rate of cancer cell growth by 5 percent at both doses. This kind of investigation merits further clinical trials for using resveratrol as a colon cancer–preventive agent.

A 2012 study (Zhu et al.) revealed some interesting cancer-preventive potential from resveratrol supplementation. Thirty-nine adult women at increased breast cancer risk were randomized in a double-blind fashion to placebo, 5 milligrams, or 50 milligrams of trans-resveratrol twice daily for twelve weeks. Breast tissue from the women who received the trans-resveratrol had a decrease in methylation of a tumor suppressor gene (BRCA1). Decreased methylation has the effect of activating the tumor suppressor gene, thereby exerting more protective effects against cancer development. A 2012 pilot study (Howells et al.) looked at a novel compound, micronized resveratrol, given as 5 grams daily for fourteen days, to patients with colorectal cancer and liver metastases scheduled to undergo liver surgery. This study found resveratrol in the removed liver tissue and also found that the rate of apoptosis (programmed cell death) was significantly increased by 39 percent in malignant hepatic tissue following resveratrol treatment compared with tissue from the placebo-treated patients.

Although we don't put resveratrol in the same category as green tea and curcumin, it is emerging as an important flavonoid. The majority of research on resveratrol has been done on cells or in animals, while most of the human studies have looked at the cardiovascular disease–lowering effects of resveratrol. Those human trials that have been conducted in the area of cancer prevention, while fewer in number, collectively demonstrate strong anticancer potential. Previous concerns that resveratrol is not well absorbed or does not stay in the system long enough to have therapeutic value have been refuted by small human studies showing that up to 70 percent is absorbed and that metabolites stay in the system for as long as nine hours after ingestion.

Finding the Best Supplement. Although there are only a few clinical safety trials involving resveratrol, it appears to be nontoxic. The only consistent side effect is diarrhea. The diarrhea is not from the resveratrol, however, but from emodin, an additive some manufacturers use for anti-inflammatory actions that is known to cause diarrhea and cramping. When selecting a resveratrol product, look for one that lists the amount of emodin and resveratrol. Generally, a supplement with 90 percent or more resveratrol does not contain significant quantities of emodin. Supplements with 50 percent resveratrol usually have greater amounts of emodin and may cause diarrhea at higher doses. An effective daily dose may be 100 to 500 milligrams, best taken with food.

Theoretically, high intakes of resveratrol from supplements could increase the risk of bleeding when taken with anticoagulant and antiplatelet drugs, such as warfarin (Coumadin), clopidogrel (Plavix), and dipyridamole (Persantine) or nonsteroidal anti-inflammatory drugs (NSAIDs); however, this has not been confirmed in the scientific literature. Resveratrol may also affect the metabolism of other medications, so it is important to consult with a qualified integrative health care practitioner or pharmacist for guidance.

Antioxidants

Taking antioxidants is the fourth action step of the Five to Thrive Plan supplement strategy. Although diet should be your major source of antioxidants, it can be difficult to obtain enough antioxidants to meet the oxidative challenge of daily living. We live in a world of oxidative stress. We are exposed to many of the more than one hundred thousand chemicals in regular use through the air we breathe, the water we drink, and the materials and products we come in contact with. In fact, the vast majority of us have environmental chemicals in our body tissues, and these chemicals are reactive and destructive. Accumulation of these toxic compounds plays a role in the development of most chronic diseases, including cancer. Our bodies are designed to generate antioxidants to combat oxidants we are exposed to on a daily basis. The most important internal antioxidant, glutathione, is found in every cell in the body—in large measure to neutralize the oxidative damage of daily living. Unfortunately, with the added burden of environmental toxins, it is far too easy to overwhelm the body's antioxidant defenses. This can leave cells susceptible to damage that ultimately leads to disease, cancer included.

So how do these important antioxidants work? Antioxidants bind to toxins so they can be safely eliminated. When an oxidative reactive molecule—called a free radical—encounters an antioxidant, it is neutralized. Antioxidants trigger defensive mechanisms inside damaged cells. If a cell has undergone extensive oxidative damage, particularly to its DNA, the cell must either repair itself or, if the damage is too great, undergo apoptosis (cell suicide). Many antioxidants stimulate cell repair and apoptosis. Antioxidants support and enhance the health of all five key pathways of the body, and in so doing, they are an important part of a cancer-prevention supplement strategy.

The Positive Influence of Antioxidants

KEY PATHWAY	BENEFITS
The Immune System	• Activate cytotoxic immune cells: Glutathione stimulates the activity of cytotoxic T cells. • Reduce infections: Antioxidants reduce susceptibility to infections and promote faster healing time from infections, due in part to stimulating immune cell activity.
Inflammation	• Reduce oxidative cell damage: Antioxidants quench oxidative molecules, preventing oxidative cellular damage that, if otherwise left unchecked, triggers the activation of inflammatory genes. • Reduce markers of inflammation: Supplementation with antioxidants reduces C-reactive protein, a marker of inflammation.
Hormonal Balance	• Support thyroid and adrenal glands. The thyroid gland and the hypothalamic-pituitary-adrenal axis are dependent upon antioxidant coenzyme Q10 (CoQ10) status. • Reduce stress-induced increases in cortisol: A 2001 randomized placebo control trial (Peters et al.) found that ultramarathon runners who received 1,500 milligrams of vitamin C per day had lowered levels of adrenal stress hormone and inflammatory interleukins when compared to those runners who received 500 milligrams or less of vitamin C per day.
Insulin Resistance	• Lower glucose levels after carbohydrate intake: Insulin resistance is, in many respects, the result of oxidative damage to the insulin receptor. This is why people who are overweight and have high levels of fat-soluble toxins have an increased risk of developing insulin resistance and diabetes over their overweight counterparts with lower toxin loads. Therefore, antioxidants (particularly glutathione), by reducing oxidative damage from stored toxins, reduces insulin resistance and diabetes risk even in overweight individuals.

KEY PATHWAY	BENEFITS
Insulin Resistance, *continued*	• Lower the formation of advanced glycation endproducts (AGEs): AGEs are formed in insulin-resistant individuals and contribute to inflammation. Antioxidants reduce the formation of AGEs in insulin-resistant individuals. • Lower lipid peroxidation in diabetics: Oxidative stress plays a major role in pathogenesis of diabetes. Diabetics who supplement with antioxidants have reduced indicators of oxidation, specifically lipid peroxidation.
Digestion and Detoxification	• Preserve intestinal integrity: Antioxidants preserve the health of the intestinal mucosa, maintain sufficient secretion of digestive enzymes, and promote proper bowel function. • Support liver detoxification: The first phase of liver detoxification naturally generates oxidants. Antioxidants are used to bind and eliminate these oxidative compounds that emerge.

Cancer-Prevention Effects: Antioxidants

The importance of antioxidants in cancer prevention cannot be overstated. After all, antioxidants are the main mechanism of action in most of the cancer–prevention research regarding diet. There is a role for supplemental antioxidants in cancer prevention. An observational trial in 2012 (Greenlee et al.) examined 2,264 women who had been diagnosed with early stage, primary breast cancer and enrolled in the study, on average, two years after their diagnosis. The study found that antioxidant supplement use after diagnosis was high (81 percent of women) and that frequent use of vitamin C and vitamin E was associated with a 27 percent decreased risk of breast cancer recurrence.

Conversely, frequent use of combination carotenoids was associated with 107 percent increased risk of death from breast cancer. Supplemental carotenoids are generally associated with increased cancer risk and should be avoided as a supplement, but they are safe when consumed as a part of food. Another study published in 2012 (Gifkins et al.) evaluated the role of antioxidant intake on endometrial (uterine) cancer risk in 417 women who developed endometrial cancer and in 395 women without endometrial cancer. The study found a 38 percent decreased risk in the group with the highest total antioxidant intake compared with the lowest.

Not all antioxidants are created equal, and in the case of cancer prevention, the most important antioxidants are glutathione and CoQ10. Glutathione is critical for elimination of environmental pollutants, which lowers all types of cancer risk. CoQ10 is associated with decreased risk of cancers of the breast and thyroid as well as melanoma. Vitamin C is associated with lower risk of gastric cancer. Vitamin E and selenium, although important antioxidants, have not been shown in clinical studies to decrease cancer risk. Certainly there are other antioxidants that show promise as well; however, it is our goal to help you prioritize the ones that will influence as many of your body's pathways as possible and have strong scientific substantiation.

Finding the Best Supplement: Antioxidants (Glutathione)

Oral glutathione has been shown in clinical trials to create antioxidant effects systemically. It is absorbed intact, is broken down into its three amino acids (glutamic acid, cysteine, and glycine), and is then reassembled in the target organs or is used up by the intestinal cells themselves. However, not all oral glutathione supplements are created equal. We recommend the Setria brand ingredient as an efficient way to replenish depleted glutathione stores. This is a high-quality and nontoxic ingredient that is found in several dietary supplements. Look for it on the label of any product containing glutathione. A 250 to 500 milligram dose of glutathione in the morning is optimal, because our glutathione levels are at their lowest level in the morning. It is also possible to raise intracellular glutathione by taking nutrients that the body uses to make glutathione. These nutrients include alpha lipoic acid, selenium, and n-acetyl cysteine. Please note that if you have been diagnosed with cancer or are undergoing active treatment you should consult with an integrative practitioner before taking glutathione.

CoQ10, or ubiquinone, is also available as a supplement. Some cholesterol-lowering drugs, particularly statins, have been shown to lower blood levels of CoQ10, so people taking these medications should also take CoQ10. There are no known contraindications to taking CoQ10, though it can sometimes cause mild nausea and diarrhea, especially at doses above 200 milligrams. CoQ10 is best absorbed when taken with a meal. Typically 30 to 100 milligrams is sufficient for prevention purposes. Unfortunately, CoQ10 products can be adulterated with a fake CoQ10 compound. Make sure the CoQ10 product you are using has been tested for adulteration. To prevent oxidation, use a branded CoQ10 ingredient such as Kaneka QH, a reduced form of CoQ10.

Vitamin D

Let's wrap up this list of the Five to Thrive Plan's dietary supplements with a little sunshine—the sunshine vitamin, that is. There are numerous studies highlighting the importance of vitamin D to our health. Vitamin D_3 is a fat-soluble vitamin produced by the body. This production starts when the skin is exposed to sunlight. Vitamin D is also found in foods such as fish and fish oil (especially cod liver oil), eggs, and fortified milk. Vitamin D is a hormonal vitamin, meaning there are receptors for vitamin D in the body. In fact, every cell has vitamin D receptors on its surface. When vitamin D binds to these receptors, various processes are initiated in our cells that translate into a variety of actions.

Although we don't understand the role of vitamin D in every organ, we know that it is necessary for maintaining the body's blood and bone levels of calcium and phosphorus. Vitamin D deficiency results in increased bone loss and increases the rate of falls and fracture, especially in the elderly. Vitamin D supports immune function, and deficiency results in more colds and flu.

Vitamin D promotes cell maturation and regulates inflammation, and deficiency increases the risk of cancer and autoimmune disease. Vitamin D is used in the production of neurotransmitters in the brain and deficiency is linked to depression. The role of vitamin D in maintaining the health of each of the body's five key pathways is powerful.

The Positive Influence of Vitamin D

KEY PATHWAY	BENEFITS
The Immune System	• Suppresses autoimmunity: Immune cells activate vitamin D and express the vitamin D receptor on their surfaces. Vitamin D affects the activity of all immune cells—T cells, B cells, and antigen-presenting cells (dendritic cells and macrophages). The overall effect of vitamin D on the immune system is to suppress autoimmune reactivity.
Inflammation	• Anti-inflammatory: Deficiency of vitamin D increases the risk of almost all inflammatory diseases. Vitamin D deficiency is linked with increased inflammatory cytokines, specifically CRP, IL-6, and TNF-α. • Inhibits inflammatory cytokines: Vitamin D has been shown to inhibit the influx of inflammatory cytokines in distressed tissues.
Hormonal Balance	• Steroidal hormone: The effects of vitamin D in the body are hormonal ones, and as with other hormones, there are receptors in cells for vitamin D. Vitamin D influences bone density via hormone-like signaling. • Exerts antidepressant actions: Vitamin D insufficiency is also linked with anxiety and depression.
Insulin Resistance	• Vitamin D deficiency is linked with insulin resistance: Low blood levels of vitamin D are associated with metabolic syndrome. Obese individuals with low vitamin D levels are at increased risk for developing insulin resistance.
Digestion and Detoxification	• Gut homeostasis: Vitamin D plays an important role in gut homeostasis and in signaling between the bacteria in our digestive tract and our tissues. • Maintains healthy gut bacteria: Vitamin D is essential to maintaining healthy bacteria in the digestive tract.

Cancer-Prevention Effects: Vitamin D

Most of our vitamin D comes from exposure to sunlight. However, this source is compromised at northern latitudes and during the fall and winter months. Sunscreens and clothing also prevent vitamin D from entering our bodies. Skin-derived synthesis of vitamin D varies from person to person depending upon the pigmentation of the skin, age, sunscreen use, and amount of skin exposed to the sun. Vitamin D deficiency is more common among African Americans than Caucasians, for instance, because of greater pigmentation of darker skin. Obese people tend to be more vitamin D–deficient than nonobese individuals. Vitamin D levels are compromised in people with inflammatory digestive diseases and in people with dysbiosis (imbalanced gut bacteria), because they are not able to efficiently absorb vitamin D from dietary sources. There are also some individuals with inherited genetic alterations in their vitamin D receptors (vitamin D receptor polymorphism), which impairs their response to vitamin D, leaving them at increased risk for vitamin D deficiency conditions. This genetic polymorphism can be tested and, if present, will significantly elevate the requirements for vitamin D.

Vitamin D insufficiency, which may or may not be accompanied by symptoms, is linked to several health problems, including cancer. The role of vitamin D insufficiency in cancer development is emerging as an important rationale for vitamin D testing and remediation of deficiencies with vitamin D supplementation. Vitamin D has been examined in many large population studies that demonstrate that people with the lowest levels of vitamin D are at increased risk for developing cancers of the colon, breast, prostate, and pancreas as well as non-Hodgkins lymphoma. Even more alarming is the fact that many of these studies have shown that vitamin D insufficiency is linked with higher cancer fatality.

Fortunately, the converse is true as well. A 2007 trial (Lappe et al.) of more than a thousand healthy postmenopausal women was conducted over four years showing that women who took 1,500 milligrams of calcium with 1,100 IU of vitamin D had a lower incidence of all types of cancer compared to the women who took a placebo. Another double-blind, randomized controlled trial published in 2009 (Protiva et al.) showed that adults who took 800 IU of vitamin D daily had more apoptotic (cell death) gene expression in the colon compared to those who took a placebo. This study determined that although vitamin D and calcium were effective at increasing apoptosis, vitamin D was the most effective. A 2007 meta-analysis (Gorham et al.) concluded that higher blood levels of vitamin D were associated with a 50 percent lower risk of colorectal cancer. The authors further concluded that daily intake of 1,000 to 2,000 IU of vitamin D_3 could reduce the incidence of colorectal cancer with minimal risk.

A 2007 review (Garland et al.) of several studies on colon, ovarian, and breast cancer found that maintaining blood levels of vitamin D at or above 42 nanograms per milliliter (ng/mL) would result in prevention of 30 percent of breast cancers. Women with a history of breast cancer should certainly pay attention to their vitamin D levels, as low vitamin D levels have been associated with a faster progression of metastatic breast cancer. To make this even more significant, vitamin D insufficiency is more common among women with previously diagnosed breast cancer. This same study found that nearly 38 percent of women were deficient and nearly 39 percent were insufficient, which means that a combined 76 percent—or two-thirds of all women with a history of breast cancer—may require increased vitamin D. It doesn't take much to alter this risk. In a large population study of Mexican women published in 2012 (Fedirko et al.) an increase in serum vitamin D (measured as active vitamin D, or 25[OH]D) from less than 20 ng/mL (deficient) to above 30 ng/mL lowered the risk of breast cancer by 47 percent in premenopausal and postmenopausal women.

Prostate cancer has also been linked to vitamin D insufficiency. A 2007 study (John, Koo, and Schwartz) found that frequent recreational sun exposure in adulthood was associated with a 53 percent reduced risk of fatal prostate cancer. Other studies have confirmed that low blood levels of vitamin D are linked with increased incidence of prostate cancer and increased progression. In a thirteen-year-long study of more than nineteen thousand men in Finland (Ahonen et al.), low vitamin D (less than 16 ng/mL) was associated with a 70 percent increased rate of prostate cancer. A group of people who are at uniquely increased risk for cancer are those who have had an organ transplant and are on posttransplant immune-suppressive medications (so that they don't reject the transplanted organ). In a clinical trial published in 2012 (Obi et al.), 218 transplant recipients were followed for three years. Supplementation with vitamin D significantly lowered the risk of posttransplant malignancy by 75 percent. This study suggests the importance of vitamin D, particularly in immunosuppressed individuals, as a cancer-preventive agent.

Finding the Best Supplement: Vitamin D

There is considerable debate among practitioners and researchers about the proper and optimal vitamin D dosage. Some have suggested that amounts as high as 10,000 IU each day are safe and necessary. This dose is based on the fact that whole-body sunlight exposure can result in at least 10,000 IU per day of vitamin D. However, such a high dose has not been demonstrated to be safe. When our skin is exposed to sunlight, many different vitamin D metabolites are created that regulate each other. When we take such a high dose, this regulation is not available, so oral intake is very different than high intake from the sun.

For decades, it was assumed that 400 IU of vitamin D was sufficient. Today that is considered too low for the majority of adults. Researchers, health care practitioners, and large institutional organizations now agree that most adults who have insufficient vitamin D levels will require at least 800 IU daily. Most researchers and practitioners have targeted 1,200 IU to 2,000 IU daily as an optimal dosage range needed to increase vitamin D into the normal range. Long-term dosage of 2,000 IU daily has been shown in a variety of studies to be safe and well tolerated. Doses higher than this should only be consumed under the guidance of a health care practitioner. Your practitioner will measure your blood level of vitamin D to help determine your optimal dosage and will use your vitamin D test along with other parameters of your health to determine if your dosage is appropriate. Health care practitioners can also guide you to reliable vitamin D products. Vitamin D should be used with caution in patients taking the heart medication digoxin, because the combination can cause elevated blood calcium levels which, in turn, may cause abnormal heart rhythms.

Keep in mind, getting some time in the sun (but not in excess) is an excellent way to increase vitamin D levels. If you expose your arms and legs or your hands, arms, and face to sunlight for five to fifteen minutes two to three times each week

Disclosure Statement

As you will notice, we have mentioned a few specific brands of supplement ingredients. It is important to note that we are not paid spokespeople for any of the brands mentioned in this book. We recommend branded ingredients when we are aware of compelling advantages, significant research, or superior quality. We recommend ingredients and brands we trust. However, two of the ingredient suppliers we recommend in the book do support our Five to Thrive educational initiative (fivetothriveplan.com) and those are Kyowa Hakko (Setria) and Taiyo International (Suntheanine and Sunphenon).

between 10:00 a.m. and 3:00 p.m. during the spring, summer, and fall months, you should have sufficient vitamin D levels without getting sunburned. If you are in the sun for more than fifteen minutes, wear sunscreen. Of course, if you are very fair-skinned or have a history of skin cancer, limit your sun exposure completely. That said, for the majority of us, some sun is not dangerous and is in fact good for us.

The Importance of Individualization

In this chapter we've used the body's five key pathways and the concept of epigenetics to help you prioritize your supplement choices. Gaining as much information as you can and individualizing your approach is the best option of all. You don't have to do that alone. Naturopathic doctors, holistic medical doctors, integrative nurse practitioners, chiropractors, holistic dieticians, nutritionists, and many pharmacists can help you. There are many qualified providers with training in dietary supplements who can guide you to making the most effective, safe, and individualized choices.

Remember, the Five to Thrive Plan's featured dietary supplements provide a great foundation, but don't limit yourself to just those. Here is a short list of supplements that can provide additional support to each of the body's key pathways:

- **The immune system.** Mushrooms, such as *Trametes versicolor* (turkey tail), *Grifola frondosa* (maitake), *Lentinula edodes* (shiitake), *Ganoderma lucidum* (reishi); yeast-derived beta-glucan; zinc; *Andrographis paniculata* (Indian echinacea); and *Astragalus membranaceus* (milk vetch).

- **Inflammation.** Cocoa flavonoids, ellagic acid, *Boswellia serrata* (Indian frankincense), tocotrienols, *Ocimum tenuiflorum* (holy basil), *Zingiber officinale* (ginger), anthocyanins, delphinidin, and quercetin.

- **Hormonal balance.** Genistein, phosphatidylserine, homeopathics, 5-hydroxy tryptophan, *Actea racemosa* (black cohosh), and *Withania somnifera* (ashwaghanda).

- **Insulin resistance.** Magnesium, B vitamins, soluble fiber, chromium, and *Gymnema sylvestre* (gurmarbooti).

- **Digestion and detoxification.** Herbal bitters, digestive enzymes, *Silybum marianum* (milk thistle), glycine, spirulina, and selenium.

Thrive Thought

Think about a big solid tree with a vast trunk and a canopy of branches. As a metaphor, dietary supplements are the leaves dancing in the sunlight, diet is the roots of the tree—anchoring it deep within the ground—activity are the branches that stretch and sway in the wind, your spirit is the force within the tree that allows it to defy gravity and reach toward the sky, and your rejuvenation are the buds that so miraculously appear every springtime. This wonderful manifestation of nature will thrive only when all are present. Much in the same way, your health will be optimized with diet, activity, dietary supplements, spirit, and rejuvenation so that you too can reach toward the sky and smile into the sun.

Simple Steps to Supplement Success

Dietary supplements are an important tool of modern health care, and they are a critical component of the Five to Thrive Plan. Try some of these simple steps to improve your health.

Be honest with your doctor. While billions of Americans take dietary supplements, more than half do not disclose this use to their doctors. Because supplements can interact with medications, you should always inform all of your health care providers about your supplement usage.

Consider the quality. One of the reasons we mentioned specific ingredients in some cases in our previous discussions of supplements is because those ingredients have been used in clinical studies. When buying supplements, don't always buy the cheapest product you find. Focus on the reputation and quality commitment of the manufacturer. In some cases, you may have to pay more, but you will be more apt to get the results you are looking for.

Remember that supplements are supplements. Don't ever think that taking supplements will replace eating a healthful diet and getting plenty of physical activity, because they won't. They are meant to *supplement* all of your other health-promoting strategies.

CHAPTER 5

Core Strategy #5:

Create Rejuvenation

While the fear of the suffering, pain, expense, and ill health that cancer can bring can be initially motivating, these fears are not sufficient to keep us engaged in living a preventive lifestyle long term. It's not enough to simply want to prevent cancer. We need to want to live life with vitality. Acknowledging risk of recurrence as a way to motivate healthy changes is important, but excessive anxiety is not helpful. Managing anxiety and finding a deeper well to support your motivation is critical to finding health and rejuvenation after cancer. The strongest sustaining factor—at the very core of our being—is our desire to feel fully alive. This ability to rejoice in life is something that for many does not come easily. Sometimes, it even takes a diagnosis of cancer to give a person the opportunity to rediscover his or her most profound desire to be alive.

If we consider life as a gift of enormous value, unique in all of creation, and of the most intricate design, then we are apt to care for this gift with reverence. Embarking upon a lifestyle that supports health and vitality becomes more than a list of things to try to do better. All of a sudden, these diet changes, exercise programs, and dietary supplements become guideposts lighting the way toward complete immersion in the richness of living. It is this profound sense of being alive that we hope to inspire. To do this, we need to find ways to instill deep rejuvenation as a part of our routines.

Rejuvenation and the Five Key Pathways

Living a rejuvenated life, in addition to giving you renewed joy, also positively impacts your physical well-being. Rejuvenation definitely supports the health of the five key pathways, while stress negatively impacts them.

The Immune System

Regular relaxation is one of the best ways to improve immunity. A 2011 clinical trial (Kang et al.) found that relaxation and relaxation-specific practices, even practiced as infrequently as ten minutes twice a month over a ten-month period of time, improved immunity in women with recently diagnosed breast cancer. Specifically, NK cell activity and white blood cell count improved.

Inflammation

Caregivers have some of the highest stress levels of any group of people. Research has shown that caregivers have increased gene expression of pro-inflammatory genes—namely, NF-kappaB, C-reactive protein, and IL-1. The constant and severe stress of caregiving epigenetically influences genes that make inflammatory compounds. When these genes are activated to produce these compounds, the risk for inflammatory diseases such as cancer and heart disease increases. Stress reduction is crucial for all of us, but especially important for caregivers.

Hormonal Balance

Several studies have shown that night-shift workers have an increased risk of developing some cancers, specifically hormone-dependent cancers such as breast and prostate. The reason is that shift work can disrupt the body's natural sleep cycle and therefore disrupt key hormonal body systems. A study published in 2012 (Hansen and Lassen) showed that female night-shift workers were 40 percent more likely to develop breast cancer than women who worked daytime hours. A 2012 study (Parent et al.) demonstrated that men who work the night shift are nearly three times more likely to develop prostate cancer.

Insulin Resistance

Several studies have demonstrated that lack of sleep increases insulin resistance, which is a risk factor for many illnesses, including diabetes and cancer. A 2010 study (Donga et al.) demonstrated that even just one night of partial sleep deprivation (fewer than four hours) induced signs of insulin resistance. Years of getting fewer than six hours of sleep each night induces insulin resistance and is associated with obesity and diabetes. When we are sleep-deprived, we disrupt the daily circadian rhythm that controls blood sugar balance, and we can lose insulin sensitivity. Our bodies are simply not programmed to manage our blood sugar levels on insufficient sleep. Getting enough rest will help avoid insulin resistance.

Digestion and Detoxification

The balancing part of our autonomic nervous system, sympathetic activity, is often referred to as our flight-or-fight response. When we are faced with stress, our heart rate increases, pupils dilate, blood vessels open wider, and breathing increases. If we are under continual stress, we have increased sympathetic activity and decreased parasympathetic activity.

One result of this state is that the digestive system does not receive sufficient stimulation. Over time, this will compromise the regularity of bowel movements, which in turn will affect the type and quantity of bacteria in our intestines. Imbalanced bacteria and altered bowel regularity will disrupt the integrity of the intestines—possibly leading to leaky gut syndrome, which facilitates the absorption of toxins from the intestines into the blood. These toxins require detoxification by the liver, and if copious amounts are released, it can overwhelm the liver detoxification pathway. When this happens, our cells are left vulnerable to carcinogens that are normally detoxified.

Finding ways to relax and cope with stress is essential. There are many ways to discover a deep sense of rejuvenation. For example, in the middle of a busy day, find a comfortable seat near a window where the early afternoon sunshine is streaming in and simply close your eyes and let yourself feel the warmth and coziness of the sun's rays. You can experience this profound sense of gratitude for life by inhaling that first aroma of freshly brewed coffee in the morning and cherishing the anticipation of the first sip. Reaching out for a loved one's hand and clasping it in yours is another simple yet profound connection to life. It is these brief moments that both remind us and allow us to experience the deeply rooted joy of life. Pausing and recognizing the frequency of these moments, and then artfully stringing them together, helps us create our rejuvenated living landscape.

Five Critical Action Steps

In the Five to Thrive rejuvenation strategy, we highlight five critical action steps that we aptly call the Five Rs of Rejuvenation. By focusing on these steps, you will be able to create a sense of ongoing vitality and fulfillment. As humans, we ultimately require no instruction on how to surrender into forgiveness or living life in awe. However, there are some action steps that make it easier to bring these attributes into our daily lives. These steps form the foundation of the Five to Thrive rejuvenation strategy.

1. Rhythm

2. Rest

3. Relax

4. Replenish

5. Remediate

Each of these concepts helps facilitate the ability to experience our lives fully and completely. These Five Rs create a significant sense of wellness on a psychological/emotional/spiritual level, but also on the physical plane. The Five Rs are powerful change agents that optimize the health of each of the body's five key pathways. Let's delve a little deeper into each one.

Rhythm

In large part, our bodies function in accordance with built-in rhythms that are dictated by the natural world around us. These are called circadian rhythms, and they influence our bodily functions in a patterned way each day. These daily rhythms are driven by an internal clock, which responds to the change from day to night. This central timekeeping system is located in the brain and is synchronized to daylight through photoreceptors in the eyes. Time-related messages are sent out as hormones that circulate throughout the body and as electrical signals that travel along our nerves, sending messages to cells and organs. These hormonal and nerve messages sync secondary clocks found within our cells to our central clock. In this way, our bodies stay in rhythm with the world around us.

The most obvious example of circadian rhythms is our natural wakefulness during the day and our sleepiness at night. This is due, in part, to the nighttime stimulation of melatonin. Melatonin is a hormone secreted by the pineal gland in the brain.

It causes us to feel sleepy and suppresses the activity of many cellular functions, enabling our bodies to rest. Our wakefulness during the day begins as our eyes are exposed to morning light. This triggers a shutdown of melatonin production. At the same time, early in the morning, the level of certain wakefulness hormones, such as cortisol from the adrenal gland, rises. Cortisol follows a daily pattern, reaching its highest level in the morning and lowest in the evening.

Many other bodily functions, including the five key pathways emphasized throughout the Five to Thrive Plan, are under the influence of this internal timekeeping system. This rhythmic influence is so strong that if we become disconnected from our innate clock—for instance, if we work the night shift or stay up into the early hours of the morning and then sleep during the day—our immune cells, for example, are much less efficient at recognizing threats and destroying invaders. Altered circadian rhythms reduce our resistance to environmental stressors, accelerating oxidative and inflammatory damage. People with impaired circadian rhythms develop digestive insufficiency, may experience constipation or diarrhea, and may develop changes in the bacterial balance in the digestive tract. Disrupting our circadian rhythm by becoming out of sync with the normal cycle of day and night will over time impair each of the body's five key pathways. The net result of this disarray over time can be the development of cancer. Thus, the health impact of regaining normal circadian rhythms cannot be overstated.

For most of us, this is as simple as retraining ourselves to go to sleep soon after it becomes dark and to wake with the beginning of daylight. The artificial lights we have in modern society have enabled us to experience very long days and short nights. While it may not be possible to go to bed at eight every night and wake up at six in the morning, it should be possible for most people to adjust their schedules to facilitate more sleep when it's dark and more activity when it's light. Even after several weeks of this schedule, one's circadian rhythm will regain its synchronicity, and with this, health will improve. If you have a schedule that is out of sync with your internal clock, it is typically helpful to make adjustments in small increments. The importance of establishing consistent rhythms is vital and well worth the retraining effort. Although deviations from your normal schedule will happen from time to time, the occasional late night will not unravel the health benefits that you have gained as long as most of your days are lived in the right rhythm—activity in daylight and sleeping at nighttime.

Rest

We should get eight hours of sleep each night, yet more than a third of Americans sleep six hours or fewer. Furthermore, some people who get sufficient hours of sleep are not getting high-quality sleep. The 2002 National Sleep Foundation Sleep in America poll (Kryger et al.) found that approximately 15 percent of people in the United States suffer from a sleep disorder. The most common sleep disorder is insomnia, defined as difficulty falling asleep, frequent nighttime waking, and not feeling refreshed in the morning. The link between lack of sleep and poor health is getting stronger. Insufficient sleep—either in amount or quality—impacts each of the body's five key pathways.

Many clinical studies have shown that lack of sleep (fewer than eight hours a night) can reduce the strength of the immune system, create a chronic inflammatory state, disrupt hormonal activity, cause insulin resistance, and impede optimal digestive and detoxification function. For this reason, sufficient sleep is a must. Unfortunately, there are many factors that can interfere with the quality of our sleep. These include unresolved stress, a noisy bedroom environment, too much light in the bedroom, a bedroom that is too warm, hormonal issues such as hot flashes, too much alcohol, insufficient protein in the evening meal, and side effects from medications. If you are having trouble getting a good night's rest, it is important to survey your life to see what might be causing the trouble. In addition to looking at these issues, try these tips to get a good night's rest:

- Keep your bedroom dark, cool, and quiet.
- Exercise daily to prevent pent-up energy from keeping you awake.
- Eat protein at dinnertime so your blood sugar remains better balanced over the night; some people experience poor sleep because drops in blood sugar wake them.
- Consider taking dietary supplements such as L-theanine (Suntheanine), valerian, chamomile, lavender, 5-HTP, homeopathic remedies, or melatonin.

It is best to seek advice from a qualified health care practitioner before starting on these supplements to avoid any interactions with other medications or other unintended side effects. If you are experiencing difficulties with sleep, talk to a health care professional about your options. Getting the proper amount of rest each day is absolutely critical to your health. If you are considering taking sleeping pills to remedy your insomnia, here is a word of caution: a large study published in 2012 (Kripke, Langer, and Kline) demonstrated that there was a 35 percent higher risk of developing cancer in people who chronically took prescription sleeping pills like Ambien, Restoril, and others. Even people in the study who only took one or two sleeping pills a month had an increased risk of dying sooner than those who did not take any sleeping pills. It is important to work with an integrative or naturopathic physician to explore natural ways to ease insomnia and other sleep problems.

Relax

In addition to getting enough sleep, finding ways to unwind is a great way to feel rested and restored. Relaxation is different from rest but just as essential. Rest is tied more directly to the physical act of sleeping and resting, while relaxation is a state of well-being. In many ways, relaxation is the opposite of stress. When we allow ourselves to feel relaxed, we let go of feelings of stress, anxiety, and depression. We facilitate the body's ability to regain internal homeostasis (balance). Relaxation serves the critical role of creating the time and space needed to restore mental and emotional balance. Unfortunately, the pace of modern living is somewhat antithetical to relaxation. Most of us are working long hours, perhaps raising a family, and usually multitasking.

One thing that can prevent us from relaxing is feeling anxiety. Many people have some level of anxiety most of the time. Research has shown that anxiety is actually a manifestation of the body's defense against stress. When we feel anxious, our stress response system—namely, the hypothalamic-pituitary-adrenal (HPA) axis—responds by secreting cortisol, epinephrine, norepinephrine, and interleukins. These chemicals influence many other key bodily functions. Another effect of these compounds is to alter brain activity and neurotransmitter production in a way that favors a state of anxiety. This makes sense if you think about the fact that when we encounter stress, it's natural for us to feel anxious in order to create discomfort, which in turn motivates us to move away from the stress. However, experiencing chronic anxiety can be very disruptive to overall health. People who are chronically anxious tend to eat poorly, don't exercise, and can't sleep well. Anxious people also tend to drink more alcohol. None of these behaviors is conducive to healthful living. Not to mention the fact that chronic anxiety is itself a form of distress. If unresolved, this distress will create a generalized sense of loss of control. When we feel out of control, it can become very difficult to summon the inner resources necessary to proactively engage in a healthy lifestyle.

Relaxation is the antidote to anxiety. The path to relaxation is different for each person. Whether it comes from taking a walk in the woods, playing a musical instrument, spending time with a friend over a cup of tea, receiving a therapeutic massage, or meditating, the end result will be the same. The most important thing is to figure out what relaxes you and then prioritize that activity so you experience relaxation every day. Make a list of five things that help you relax, then make a commitment to do one of those five things every day. Before you begin your day, ask yourself, how am I going to relax today? Then be sure to schedule that relaxing activity just as you would an important meeting. In our type-A society, relaxation and downtime can be frowned upon. People who are not busy all of the time may be seen as unproductive loafers. Nothing could be further from the truth. People who engage in regular relaxation are actively building their health. Health does not happen in the background of our lives; it requires a diverse mix of ingredients, including relaxation. It's time to shed any guilt and step confidently into a life that includes regular relaxing downtime.

Replenish

The fourth R is for replenish. On one level, "replenishment" means supplying nutrients to the body for optimal functioning. Chapters 3 and 4, on diet and dietary supplements respectively, describe the essential nutrients for a comprehensive cancer-prevention plan. In this section, however, "replenishment" takes on additional meaning. To rejuvenate one's sense of health and well-being, one must replenish the components of life that have been left unattended and neglected. In addition to replenishing our physical bodies with food, sleep, and movement, our soul needs replenishing. Expressing ourselves creatively is a particularly effective way to replenish the body, mind, and soul. Several studies have shown that being creative benefits the elderly by improving mood, boosting self-esteem, and encouraging socialization. According to a 2005 article (Baikie and Wilhelm), several well-designed studies have shown that creative activity such as expressive writing can cause physiological changes that increase brain function as well as the expression of joy.

We may think of creativity as art or acting, but it's so much more. In the scientific literature, creativity is described as something that is novel yet meaningful. A comprehensive literature review published in 2010 (Stuckey and Nobel) looked at a variety of creative activities, including music, drawing, dance, and expressive writing. Many physical and emotional benefits were found, including enhanced mood, reduced pain, more energy, and even increased immune activity. The researchers found that creative artistic engagement "has significant positive effects on health." They concluded: "Through creativity and imagination, we find our identity and our reservoir of healing." In a paper published in 2005 (Baikie and Wilhelm), the authors explain that writing about traumatic, stressful, or emotional events for fifteen to twenty minutes on three to five occasions significantly improved physical or psychological outcomes. Although this study used writing as a healing method, certainly writing can be used as a creative outlet as well.

Being creative can also entail visiting museums, concert halls, craft stores, or local boutiques. It can include keeping a daily journal, doing puzzles, traveling, or joining a book club. Being creative means that you agree to put rules aside. You are coloring outside the lines, so to speak. Whatever you create is just that—something you create. You don't have to produce masterpieces, and you can discard anything that you make; the replenishment comes from the doing. Just by being open to your own creativity and the creativity of others, you will feel replenished and experience a renewed sense of playfulness.

Speaking of being playful, that's another way to replenish and recharge your inner spark. A young man came up to us after one of our talks on thriving after cancer and told us about how he had started jogging in his nearby park. As he increased his distance, he was able to jog several miles through the park to a swing set on the other side. As a reward, he decided one day to end his run with a swing on the swing set. He now makes that a part of his regular routine. "At first I thought I must look silly, a grown man swinging on the swings, but then I realized I didn't care. I felt like a kid again." Sometimes we can achieve replenishment in unsuspecting ways, and being playful can be one of the most joyous ways to do that. The best part is that being playful often involves smiling, laughing, and loving—significant ingredients to replenishment success!

Remediate

Cancer is often referred to as a harsh teacher, but it is a teacher nonetheless. One lesson it offers us is the opportunity to remediate our relationships. How do we correct, make right, or move on? To remediate is to step closer to the untended aspects of our relationships and honestly scrutinize the wounds, holes, and ill-fitting components. With this insight, we must then be willing to forgive and make needed changes. The fifth R of the rejuvenation strategy of the Five to Thrive Plan is to reevaluate relationships as well as life's priorities. The goal is to live in synchronicity with our deepest, truest aspirations, surrounded by people with whom we can exchange genuine support and express unimpeded love.

Remediation encompasses more than relationships to people; it also involves our relationship to our work, our living situation, and how we express ourselves in the world. To remediate our lives could encompass such transformations as changing careers, ending relationships, confronting a loved one, coming to terms with a part of ourselves not yet revealed, moving to a new city, or going back to school in midlife. Or remediation could mean doing small things, like leaving work early, cooking meals as a family, or making a plan to be in nature as often as you can. In some cases, being open to the reevaluation and remediation process takes courage. In all cases, it takes commitment.

Evaluating your present life situation may require asking yourself a series of questions. It may mean facing some difficult answers and decisions. Are there areas of your life that are destructive or unhealthy? Do you have toxic relationships that need to be ended or transformed? How can you become more aligned with who you are and who you want to be? Are your work, relationships, and way of living consistent with your values, passions, and aspirations? We each have a different way we manage this phase of the Five to Thrive Plan, but the important thing is to include it as a crucial part of your risk reduction plan.

A central part of remediation is forgiveness—of yourself and others. We are each imperfect beings. At times, we do things that are not kind to ourselves or to others, and we may harbor self-reproach and criticism. This judgment constricts the soul, and yet we remain imperfect. The only way out of this destructive cycle is forgiveness. Through forgiveness, we settle into our own humanity and accept the humanity in others. Forgiveness is freeing and rejuvenates us on a very deep level.

Take our personal examples: After Al Alschuler (Lise's father) was diagnosed with cancer, he lived each day as if it were his last. He traveled all over the country in a concerted effort to visit and talk with all of the significant people in his life. He wanted to heal with others and help them heal as well. He asked for forgiveness, gave forgiveness, and wisely asked if there was anything he could do to help heal old wounds and give those he loved a sense of peace. In the case of Eunice Gazella (Karolyn's mother), remediation took the form of dictated letters to her husband and six children. The individual letters expressed her love, hopes, and dreams for each person. The letters were for her as much as they were for the recipients. Her family appreciated this loving gesture and it gave her peace.

Through a process of self-evaluation and taking a good hard look at our surroundings, we can begin to live life fully, as if each day were our last. Now one might think that living each day as if it were your last would entail all forms of gluttony and immediate pleasures. Really, though, living each day as if it were our last creates an acute sense of the value, the preciousness, and the wonder of life that is contained within each moment—an appreciation that transcends the material and stems from the heart. With this deep sense of appreciation, our desires become focused on gratitude and simply finding time to reflect on life. Remediation helps us get that clarity. Al certainly had days of frustration, anger, and sadness, but he also spent an extraordinary number being deeply in love with life. This was, just as he had hoped, his greatest gift not only to his children but also to all those who cared about him. In modeling the meaning of remediation, he graciously showed those he loved the meaning of living life fully and exuberantly.

Thrive Thought

Words often used to describe rejuvenation include vigor, restoration, and freshness—all feelings we long to have. One way to help us gain these feelings is to be in touch with our personality type and how we interact with others. Are you an extrovert or introvert? Are you a pleaser, doer, or ring leader? There are great books and methods to help you get in touch with your personality type and how you interact with other personality types (some of these are listed in the Resources). However you describe yourself, recognize that understanding your personality will help you better understand how you recharge your battery for successful rejuvenation. For example, how do you feel in large groups? Are you invigorated by such interactions, or do you find that you become drained if you are around people all the time? Perhaps you require some introversion to regain your balance. Being in touch with what you need to recharge is critical, and it just may mean that sometimes you need to be alone.

Simple Steps to Enhanced Rejuvenation

Rejuvenation is about rediscovering our love of life. Within this joyful embrace resides the foundation of health and vitality. Rejuvenation is fundamental to cancer prevention and to overall health because it connects us to our sacred purpose. The foundational Five Rs—rhythm, rest, relax, replenish, and remediate—will seed vitality and sacredness in our lives so we can bloom into our every day. Try these simple steps to enhance rejuvenation:

Practice meditation. Think about several times when you felt loved and picture those times in your mind's eye. These are now your love meditations. Take some time each week to listen to relaxing music and think about the love meditations you have created. Recall how you felt, whom you were with, and how appreciated and loved you felt at that time. When you are done, take some full, deep breaths and let those moments sink into the very fabric of your being.

Speak from the heart. Think about someone whom you are angry with and consider how you can forgive him or her in order to let go of your anger. Create some time to communicate with this person—either in person or in writing—about your love and forgiveness.

Really relax. During these hectic times, even when we think we are relaxing, we may still be thinking about work, family, and other commitments. It's important to take time and really unplug fully. Even if it's just five minutes a couple of times a day, make sure those five minutes are unencumbered and free of stressful thoughts and a racing mind.

Cultivate individualized creativity. Explore, express, and enhance your creative being to help rejuvenate mind, body, and soul. You may need to think outside the box, but that too is a part of the creative process. Remember, your creative outlet is uniquely yours.

CHAPTER 6

Screening Strategies
That Make Sense

Sometimes it's easier to take care of our car, home, family, and pets than it is to take care of ourselves. Every three thousand miles we get the oil changed in the car, each winter we have the furnace looked at, we take the dog to the vet once a year, we get the kids ready for school in the fall, and we remind loved ones about important health appointments. But when it comes to our own tune-up, there is a tendency to put it on the back burner. We consistently hear two different trains of thought when it comes to going to the doctor, and they sound like this:

- I'm too busy. There's nothing wrong with me.
  I'll go next year.

- I'm afraid. What if they find something?

The first response, while perhaps true, is also an expression of denial that is simply another version of the second response. The fear expressed in the second response often comes from those who've had a previous diagnosis of cancer. We know how that feels—that sinking and shocking feeling when you hear those words "You have cancer." It's our mission to keep those words as far away from you as possible. The Five to Thrive integrative cancer-prevention plan we've described will help give you the confidence you need to work proactively with your team of health care professionals. You can transform your relationship with your doctors and the doctor visit by taking charge of your health and partnering with your health care provider for your own benefit. The plan will also give you the strength and resolve to tackle whatever is discovered along your journey.

Also, the way you handle your health has far-reaching effects. How you carry out your cancer-prevention plan will set the tone for your entire family and your network of friends. You can lead by example, allowing your actions to loudly send the right message to those you influence. Whether or not you've had a previous diagnosis, this chapter will help you create a practical, effective plan that includes proper screening and integrative health care.

We begin by addressing basic screening, tests that are designed to look for cancer before symptoms arise. The goal of screening is to rule out cancer or catch it early. Please keep in mind that if your doctor recommends a screening test, it doesn't mean that you have cancer. If your screening test is abnormal, you may have to have additional tests. These are called diagnostic tests. In addition to these screening tests, there are other laboratory tests that can better assess the status of each of your body's five key pathways (the immune system, inflammation, hormonal balance, insulin resistance, and digestion and detoxification). Although these tests are not necessarily diagnostic, they do provide an objective assessment of various parameters that indicate the status of each of the pathways. These tests are referred to as biomarker tests, functional medicine tests, or physiological assessments. We'll highlight some of these tests momentarily, but first let's review standard screening.

While everyone, particularly those with a history of cancer, should be on a regular schedule of checkups and screening tests, there are certain symptoms that indicate the need for a prompt evaluation. Although these symptoms do not necessarily mean that you have cancer, they can be signs of cancer. Cancer is always most curable when it is diagnosed early, so please take these symptoms seriously.

- Unexplained, persistent, and worsening pain
- Extreme tiredness
- Unexplained weight loss (this includes desirable weight loss but still unrelated to specific diet or exercise changes)
- Night sweats and fever
- Unexplained changes in your bowel frequency, or blood in your stool or urine
- A worsening dry cough (not associated with a cold or bronchitis)
- Unexplained and long-lasting voice hoarseness
- Skin pigmentation changes, yellowness, a bleeding mole, or itchiness

Should you develop any of these symptoms, see your doctor for a diagnostic work-up. In addition to following up on specific symptoms, it is important to activate a regular screening program. Let's look at screening for various cancers, beginning with the colon and working our way north.

Colon Cancer Screening Tests

Colon cancer screening is critical and reduces death from colon cancer by up to 80 percent.

Colonoscopy

With this test, the doctor uses a flexible tube with a miniature camera on the end to look inside the colon and rectum.

Timing and Frequency: Beginning at age fifty or earlier with a family history of colon cancer or digestive symptoms and every five to ten years thereafter.

Rationale: This test allows for visualization of the colon to identify polyps (a risk factor for cancer).

Fecal Occult Blood Test

This is a home-test that your doctor will provide to you. Two samples are collected from one to three consecutive stools, depending upon the type of stool test. The samples are applied to a specially prepared card. These cards are then analyzed by a laboratory for microscopic signs of blood.

Timing and Frequency: Beginning at age fifty and every two years thereafter.

Rationale: Noninvasive test that identifies hidden blood in the stool, which can indicate the presence of cancer, ulceration, or inflammation of the digestive tract.

Flexible Sigmoidoscopy, Double-Contrast Barium Enema, or CT Colonography (Virtual Colonoscopy)

Flexible sigmoidoscopy enables the doctor to see the sigmoid colon, which is the last one-third of the colon, whereas a colonoscopy allows the doctor to see the entire colon. With a barium enema, after a liquid is ingested, X-rays are taken of the colon and rectum. A CT colonography is also known as a virtual colonoscopy because it is a noninvasive scan of the colon.

Timing and Frequency: After your initial colonoscopy, you should have some type of testing every five years that can include these tests. Your doctor will help you determine which of these tests may be necessary, as well as timing and frequency.

Rationale: If any of these three tests is positive, a colonoscopy should be performed.

Prostate Cancer Screening Tests

Although a prostate-specific antigen (PSA) blood test is used for prostate cancer screening, an elevated PSA should not be used as the only factor in determining if cancer is present. A high PSA number should also not be used as the only reason to do biopsies or use aggressive anticancer treatments. In addition to a digital rectal exam performed by a physician, these other factors should be considered along with the PSA level:

- Size of the prostate gland
- Speed at which PSA levels are changing
- Medications that may affect PSA, such as finasteride (Proscar), dutasteride (Avodart), and even some herbal extracts such as saw palmetto
- Age

PSA Blood Test

Testing for elevated PSA in the blood is the only prostate cancer-screening blood test presently available. Prostate cancer screening is also accomplished with a digital rectal examination as a part of an annual examination.

Timing: Beginning at age fifty. PSA may be indicated before age fifty in men who are African American, have a family history of prostate cancer in any of their first-degree relatives, or have had some prostate health issues. PSA testing is not likely necessary for men over age seventy-five.

Frequency:

- Yearly PSA screening for men whose PSA level is 2.5 ng/mL to 4.0 ng/mL, or individualized depending on other health factors.
- PSA screening every two years for men whose PSA is less than 2.5 ng/mL.
- PSA greater than 4.0 ng/mL requires additional diagnostic evaluation, which may include biopsy.
- Some doctors follow guidelines that advise annual PSA testing with PSA values greater than 1.0 ng/mL.

Rationale: PSA is a protein that is produced in the prostate to help liquefy semen. Some of those proteins make their way into the bloodstream. While it's true that elevated PSA levels can indicate cancer, they can also be elevated in men who have prostatitis (inflamed prostate) or an enlarged prostate (benign prostatic hyperplasia—BPH). Conversely, PSA levels may be in the normal range even when cancer is present. The United States Preventive Services Task Force recommends against PSA screening in healthy men due to the potential risks of biopsy and treatment of non-life threatening disease outweighing the potential benefits of the screening. The frequency of PSA screening is different from man to man and should be carefully discussed with your medical provider.

Ovarian Cancer Screening Tests

In addition to testing, the following symptoms, if unexplained, should be discussed with your doctor:

- Abdominal pressure or bloating
- Changes in bowel or bladder habits
- Abdominal weight gain with clothes fitting more tightly around your waist
- Low-back pain
- Persistent indigestion, gas, or nausea
- Changes in menstruation, such as irregular or heavy bleeding

Gynecological Exam

There is no standard screening test currently available for ovarian cancer. The best way to screen for ovarian cancer is to obtain a gynecological exam. In cases of suspicious symptoms, your doctor may recommend a transvaginal ultrasound and CA-125 test.

Timing and Frequency: Gynecological exams should be scheduled annually.

Rationale: Some people confuse the tumor marker test that evaluates circulating levels of CA-125 (a protein shed into the blood from ovarian cancer cells, but also from inflamed tissues) with screening; however, this is not a routine screening test. An increased level of CA-125 in the blood can indicate cancer; however, other noncancerous conditions, such as uterine fibroids, endometriosis, and even pregnancy can increase CA-125 levels. What's more, CA-125 levels may not be increased with early-stage ovarian cancers, so they can give a false sense of security. The CA-125 test is most effectively used as a part of a diagnostic work-up and after diagnosis of ovarian cancer to track treatment success or progression of the disease.

Cervical and Uterine Cancer Screening Tests

In addition to testing, consult with your doctor if you are having any of the following symptoms:

- Unexplained pain in your lower belly or around the pelvic area
- Issues with your menstrual periods
- Vaginal discharge, itching, burning, or bad odor
- Severe cramps or other issues associated with premenstrual syndrome (PMS)
- Unexplained spotting after menopause

Pap Test and Pelvic Exam

Cervical cancer screening is done during a gynecological exam, also referred to as a pelvic exam. During the pelvic exam, your health care practitioner will conduct a Pap test. This involves swabbing the cervix to collect cells for lab testing for precancerous changes or cancer. Also, during the pelvic exam, your practitioner will conduct a bimanual exam to check other reproductive organs, such as the ovaries and uterus. A rectal exam may also be done after the bimanual exam. A urine test is done to look for signs of infection, inflammation, and cancer of the bladder.

Timing and Frequency: Annual gynecological exams begin within a couple of years after active vaginal intercourse but no later than age twenty-one. According to the American Cancer Society, beginning at age thirty, women who have had three consecutive normal Pap test results can start doing screening every two to three years rather than annually. Women who are seventy years or older and have had at least three normal Pap tests in a row and no abnormal test results within the past ten years may choose to stop having Pap tests.

Rationale: The major risk factor for cervical cancer is infection with certain strains of the human papillomavirus (HPV), a sexually transmitted virus. For this reason, testing for HPV during the pelvic exam in women who are sexually active is important. A key sign of HPV is genital warts.

Breast Cancer Screening Tests

We often hear questions about breast thermography. At this point there is not enough data to suggest that thermography can be used as a screening method for breast cancer. There is room for error in how the thermography is done, and the interpretation of the findings can vary. Until there is a certification program and guidelines for thermography testing, it should only be used in addition to the standard screenings, described below.

Mammogram

A series of radiographic (X-ray) images of the breast tissue. The breast tissue is compressed between radiographic plates to obtain the images.

Timing and Frequency: The American Cancer Society recommends an annual mammogram beginning at age forty. Based

Reducing Radiation Worries

Some screening tests—like CT scans, mammograms, MRIs, and X-rays—increase our exposure to radiation, which could theoretically increase our risk of developing cancer. Yet these are valid tests that are often necessary to help us rule out cancer or catch it early. Just before a screening test that emits radiation, loading up on antioxidants can give your cells added protection from the radiation in these scans. Although there are no clinical trials that prove protective benefit from our recommendation, there is good theoretical rationale. Plus, there is little risk of harm and no danger of interfering with the scan. If you are taking any blood-thinning or chemotherapy medications, consult with your doctor before adding these supplements—even for the short time that we are suggesting.

Here is what we recommend: Take at least three of the following nutrients three times each—approximately two hours before the scan, again within thirty minutes before the scan, and ideally within thirty minutes after the scan.

- Vitamin D = 1,000 IU each dose
- Vitamin E (mixed tocopherols and tocotrienols) = 400 IU each dose
- Glutathione (Setria brand) = 250 milligrams each dose
- N-acetylcysteine = 250 milligrams each dose
- Alpha-lipoic acid = 100 milligrams each dose
- Spirulina or blue-green algae = 2,000 milligrams each dose
- Selenium citrate or picolinate = 100 micrograms each dose (Note: Two Brazil nuts provide the same amount of selenium.)

All of these nutrients have been shown to support the detoxification pathway and increase the body's antioxidant levels, thus helping to protect cells from the damaging effects of radiation. Rather than avoiding an important test, you can enhance your body's innate protective ability—it's the best of both worlds!

on published research, the U.S. Preventive Services Task Force recommends that women begin routine mammography at age fifty, not age forty, and recommends a mammogram every two years until age seventy-four rather than annually.

Women who have a strong family history (mother or sister) of breast cancer or test positive for the BRCA gene should talk to their doctor about getting an MRI in addition to a mammogram. Breast ultrasound is another option for these women.

People with a history of breast cancer who are not experiencing any symptoms should receive an annual mammogram with or without ultrasound (or, for women in whom a mammogram did not find the original tumor, a breast MRI), along with a physical examination by their doctor every three to four months for the first three years following treatment, every six months for the next two years, and then annually after five years.

Rationale: The recommendations of the U.S. Preventive Services Task Force are based upon their findings that the benefit of starting mammograms earlier and repeating them more often did not outweigh the harm they impose—mainly unnecessary biopsies and additional radiation exposure from the mammograms.

Clinical Breast Examination

Examination and palpation of the breast tissue and axillae (armpits) by a health care provider to assess tissue irregularities.

Timing and Frequency: The American Cancer Society recommends women have a clinical breast exam (CBE), which is a breast exam done by a trained health care professional, every three years between ages twenty and thirty-nine and every year after age forty.

Breast MRI

Highly sensitive imaging of the breast tissue using magnetic resonance imaging (MRI).

Timing and Frequency: Breast MRI is utilized for women with dense breast tissue for whom a mammograph is not diagnostic. These women may be screened with breast MRI. Based on the woman's individual circumstances, the timing and frequency of the MRI will be determined by the physician.

Rationale: This is especially important for women under age fifty who are at high risk, because younger women have a tendency to have more dense breast tissue and mammography is not as sensitive with dense tissue.

Lung Cancer Screening Tests

Presently there are no routine tests done to screen for lung cancer in the general population; however, people who smoke should get a chest X-ray or chest CT scan on an annual basis. The present lung cancer screening tests are typically utilized when symptoms are present, and the goal of these tests is to rule out cancer or detect it early so it is more treatable.

Chest X-ray

This is an X-ray of the organs and bones inside the chest.

Timing and Frequency: People with a history of smoking or exposure to smokers, at minimum, need a chest X-ray annually. For nonsmokers, any persistent, dry cough should be evaluated with a chest X-ray.

Rationale: This is an inexpensive test that is easily performed. While it is not as accurate as other tests, it can still identify areas of concern.

CT Scan

This procedure uses low-dose radiation to create a series of pictures of the chest area.

Timing and Frequency: An annual chest computed tomography (CT) is the best screening tool, as it is more sensitive at finding lung tumors.

Rationale: While chest X-rays are less expensive, they are also less accurate than a CT test. Screening with CT scans reduces the rate of death from lung cancer by 20 percent.

Skin Cancer Screening Tests

Skin cancer screening is extremely important and saves countless lives. In the case of melanoma, the most serious form of skin cancer, the Skin Cancer Foundation reports that if melanoma is detected early before the tumor has spread to regional lymph nodes or other organs, the five-year survival rate is 98 percent.

Skin Examination

Here are some key things to monitor:
- Moles that have changed in appearance
- Moles that have become larger
- Moles or spots that peel, bleed, or become itchy
- New moles, sores, or abnormal-looking spots
- Ulcers or sores that do not heal

If you notice any of the above-mentioned changes, contact your doctor. If something looks abnormal, a biopsy may be required.

Timing and Frequency: Annual dermatological evaluation, particularly for those with multiple birthmarks.

Rationale: The most effective way to screen for skin cancer is by examining the skin and paying close attention to any changes.

Beyond Cancer Screening:
Biomarker Testing

Assessing the status of the body's five key pathways can potentially identify areas of function that need the most attention—we hope *before* disease develops. One way to check the status of the pathways is through biomarker tests. The biomarker tests described here all require a doctor's order and may, or may not, be covered under health insurance. The costs of the tests described vary but are generally in the one-hundred- to several-hundred-dollar range. When speaking to your doctor about ordering these tests, make sure that you know the cost of the test and whether it will be covered by insurance before agreeing to the test.

A few caveats are in order before we discuss these tests. They are not cancer diagnostic tests. These tests provide additional information that integrative, naturopathic, and chiropractic physicians may use to help them better understand how your body is functioning. Because some of these tests point to potential dysfunction, your conventional medical doctor and your oncologist may have difficulty obtaining insurance coverage for some of these tests. Some of these tests are typically outside the standard of medical practice for most conventional doctors, and therefore many oncologists and conventional doctors will not order them. To find a naturopathic physician, functional medicine doctor, or chiropractor who may be familiar with these tests, refer to the Resources at the back of the book. When you talk with your integrative doctor about these tests, it is important to recognize that all of these tests will not be ordered for you—it is the job of your integrative doctor to determine which, if any, of these tests would be helpful to provide you with the best cancer-prevention and health-optimization plan.

Although the tests described here are not exhaustive of all the tests that can be used to assess the function of the body's five key pathways, they do represent some of the more helpful ones.

Your integrative practitioner will be able to determine which tests will be most helpful and may order some of them, none of them, or may suggest additional tests for you. It is also important to emphasize that even without the results of these lab tests, you can benefit from the Five to Thrive Plan. None of these tests is required as a part of the plan.

The Immune System

Billions of immune cells are buzzing with activity inside the body every minute of every day. Assessing the overall status of this activity is not possible. However, there are attributes of immunity that we can measure to give us a snapshot of how well our defensive system is functioning, particularly its ability to protect us against potential cancer development.

White blood cell count (WBC) and differential. This count is routinely done as a part of a typical annual blood test and is a key component of follow-up blood draws in people who have had cancer. In this test, white blood cells refer to all of the immune cells in circulation. The combination of the different types of WBCs and their ratios to one another allows for the assessment of overall immune status and indicates reasons for that status.

Natural killer (NK) cell assay. This test is not routinely done but can be ordered by your doctor using a standard blood draw. The NK cell assay is a helpful way to assess innate immunity in someone with a history of cancer. Many of the immune strategies in the Five to Thrive Plan are geared to increasing NK cells and their activity. When ordered from a specialty lab, this assay also may include a functional assessment that measures the activity of NK cells.

25–OH vitamin D. This test measures blood levels of 25–OH vitamin D, which is indicative of whole body levels of vitamin D. T cells rely on vitamin D to become activated. The ideal level of serum vitamin D is not definitively known. However, many clinical studies correlate the incidence of cancers, insulin resistance, osteoporosis, cardiovascular disease, and other chronic illness when serum vitamin D is below 25 ng/mL (nanograms per milliliter). Vitamin D3 is one of the foundational dietary supplements in the Five to Thrive Plan, and it is important to assess starting blood levels of vitamin D before supplementation.

Inflammation

When inflammation exists in the body, inflamed tissue releases certain distress signals. These distress signals make their way into the blood and can be measured. These molecular signals become elevated in the blood of people with low-grade chronic inflammation. There are tests that measure these chemicals, thereby giving us an idea of underlying inflammation. Contributors to inflammation that can be measured include heavy metal exposure, food sensitivities and food allergies, pesticides, and volatile solvent exposure. Let's take a look at some of the inflammation biomarker tests.

Homocysteine. An elevated level of homocysteine is correlated with increased risk for certain cancers, such as colon cancer and breast cancer, particularly when present alongside folic acid deficiency. Elevated homocysteine is also associated with an increased risk of cardiovascular disease, neurological diseases, and autoimmune disease. Elevated homocysteine is an indirect indicator of vitamin B_{12} and folic acid levels, as deficiencies of one or both of these result in elevated homocysteine. Folic acid and vitamin B_{12} levels can be measured in the blood. Another test that can be added to B_{12} is methylmalonic acid, which can become elevated if B_{12} is deficient.

High-sensitivity (cardiac) C-reactive protein (hs-CRP). This is one of the best markers for inflammation. The hs-CRP is an acute phase protein that is released by the liver and by fat cells in response to acute inflammatory stress signals released from inflamed tissue. CRP accumulates in the blood in response to inflammation. If inflammatory signals are persistent, the level of hs-CRP will elevate in the blood.

Ferritin. Ferritin is the main cellular storage protein for iron and is concentrated in the liver and spleen. A ferritin test indirectly measures the amount of iron in your blood. Low blood levels of ferritin are an indication of iron-deficiency anemia. Elevated blood ferritin occurs with iron overload from transfusions or a disease called hemochromatosis but can also be the result of liver disease, cancer, and inflammation.

Interleukin-6. IL-6 is measured from a blood test. Tumor cells as well as cells in inflamed tissues secrete a number of molecules, including IL-6. IL-6 has a wide range of cancer-promoting actions, including activating cell division, increasing tumor blood supply, and increasing tumor invasiveness.

Interleukin-8. IL-8 is measured from a blood test. IL-8 is one of the major mediators of the inflammatory response. Macrophages, epithelial cells, and several other cell types secrete IL-8. It causes neutrophils to migrate toward the site of infection and stimulates neutrophil activity once they arrive at the site. IL-8 is also a potent angiogenic factor (stimulates blood vessel development). Cancer cells and the macrophages associated with cancerous tumors often secrete copious amounts of IL-8, which promotes pro-tumor growth cell signaling and increased blood supply to the tumor bed.

Fibrinogen. This is a clotting factor in the blood that increases with inflammation, tissue damage, insulin resistance, and some cancers. Excessive fibrinogen makes the blood too "sticky" because it is the precursor for fibrin, which is the scaffolding upon which platelets aggregate, forming clots. In addition, fibrin coats cancer cells and camouflages the cancer cells from immune system detection. Fibrin associated with cancer cells increases the development of blood vessels (angiogenesis) to the cancer.

Lipid peroxidation. Chronic and significant inflammation will stress the antioxidant reserves in the body, ultimately depleting the body's ability to mount an effective antioxidant defense. This depletion of an antioxidant defense leaves our tissues prone to oxidative, cancer-promoting damage. We can use the cells in the blood as a marker for overall oxidative stress. One such test measures the oxidative damage to the cell membranes of blood by measuring lipid peroxides.

Hormonal Balance

There are several hormonal pathways that have relevance to health and cancer risk. Blood tests can provide a snapshot of the health of this pathway. The nature of the hormonal system is to be responsive; therefore, the use and interpretation of these tests can be quite complex.

Morning cortisol. Cortisol is secreted by the adrenal gland. Cortisol levels vary considerably throughout the day so, to better standardize the results of this test, your health care provider will ask that the test be done in the morning. Elevated morning cortisol can indicate chronic or high stress but can also signal the presence of certain diseases.

DHEAs. The DHEA-sulfate test measures the amount of DHEA-sulfate, the most abundant form of DHEA, in the blood. DHEA-sulfate is a weak male hormone (androgen) produced by the adrenal gland in both men and women. DHEA is converted into testosterone, estrone, and estradiol in the adrenal glands, ovaries, and testes. DHEA-sulfate testing assesses adrenal gland function and can be helpful in conjunction with cortisol testing.

Adrenal stress index. There is a daily pattern to cortisol secretion in healthy individuals. An adrenal stress index test assesses this pattern to gain a better understanding of the dynamic function of the adrenal gland and to provide a more sensitive view into the hormonal impact of chronic stress. Typically, cortisol levels are highest early in the morning, followed by a gradual decrease to its lowest level in the late evening. Chronic stress will abnormally elevate cortisol levels and can obliterate or even reverse the normal pattern of cortisol secretion.

TSH, fT3, fT4. Thyroid function, especially low thyroid function, is associated with fatigue, weight gain, hair loss, and decreased cell repair—which is a risk factor for cancer development. Thyroid stimulating hormone (TSH) is released by the pituitary gland and when bound to its receptors on the thyroid cells, sends a message to that thyroid cell to produce thyroxine (T4). If the thyroid is under-responsive to this call to action from the pituitary, the pituitary will call louder, manifested by increased blood levels of TSH. In addition to TSH, the level of T4 and T3 (thyroid hormones) can be measured.

Estrogen profile. Estrogen is broken down by the liver into various estrogen metabolites, some of which are carcinogenic. Although the clinical value of this test is debatable, many clinicians use it to help them better understand how to support estrogen metabolism.

Insulin Resistance

Insulin resistance is considered a prediabetic condition and increases the risk for developing cancer, dementia, and cardiovascular disease. Indicators of insulin resistance, as well as insulin resistance itself, can be measured.

Blood glucose and hemoglobinA1c. Fasting blood glucose (blood sugar) is part of a standard blood chemistry test. Elevated blood sugar can diagnose diabetes, or if elevated to a lesser level, can indicate insulin resistance. HgbA1c , or glycosylated hemoglobin, is a more sensitive measure of blood sugar because it reflects the average blood sugar level over the previous eight to twelve weeks.

C-peptide. The insulin produced by your pancreas splits into two separate molecules, insulin and C-peptide. C-peptide reflects the insulin made by your pancreas. Low C-peptide levels indicate that the pancreas is not producing insulin, which can be a complication of advanced diabetes, whereas elevated C-peptide may indicate the potential for insulin resistance.

Glucose tolerance test with insulin. A more time-consuming but very accurate way to test for insulin resistance is a test available from standard conventional laboratories called the two-hour glucose tolerance test, with measurements of insulin. This test takes two hours, so bring a book! The tests starts with a blood draw for fasting blood sugar and insulin levels. Then the lab will have you drink a solution with 75 grams of sugar. You will wait for thirty minutes after consuming the drink and then a blood draw will be done to measure glucose and insulin at thirty minutes. This is repeated again at one hour from consuming the drink, and finally at two hours after consuming the drink. Dr. Mark Hyman, an expert in diabetes and functional medicine, states that simply doing a fasting and the thirty-minute insulin and glucose test may be sufficient to find most cases of insulin resistance and avoid the need to stay at the lab for the two-hour test.

Digestion and Detoxification

There are several ways to assess digestion and detoxification functioning. While you can get a good idea of how this pathway is functioning simply by paying attention to your digestion, bowel habits, and even your breath odor, additional laboratory tests such as these can be useful.

GGT. Doctors typically order gamma-glutamyl transferase (GGT) levels to determine the cause of an elevated alkaline phosphatase, another blood test. However, GGT is also a sensitive marker of exposure to persistent organic pollutants. Elevated GGT can be an indication of exposure to certain oxidative and inflammatory chemicals such as phthalates. Phthalates, or plasticizers (substances added to plastics to increase their flexibility, transparency, durability, and longevity), are found widely in consumer goods. Elevated GGT is an indirect indication of glutathione status, and if elevated, suggests a functional deficiency of antioxidative capacity—in particular, a deficiency of glutathione. Alcohol, smoking, and certain medications elevate GGT levels, so these substances must be avoided within twenty-four hours of this test in order to use it to measure environmental toxicity exposure.

Alanine transaminase (ALT). Also known as serum glutamate pyruvate transaminase (SGPT), this is part of a typical liver function test profile and is a sensitive indicator of exposure to certain chemical pollutants. Elevated ALT indicates liver damage, which in the context of known environmental exposures can indicate the presence of chemical toxicity.

Comprehensive digestive profile. This test evaluates digestion, absorption, gut flora, and the colonic environment, and evaluates for parasites. The profile is indicated for all chronic digestive problems and acute bowel pattern changes, and provides a way to better understand the microbial environment of the intestines. This test analyzes stool for digestive ability, absorption, pH, and bacterial metabolism.

Intestinal permeability. Your doctor may order an intestinal permeability test to determine the health of your intestinal lining and the potential load on your detoxification system. The lactulose and mannitol test measures the ability of these two sugar molecules to cross the intestinal lining into the blood. These sugars are not used by the body, but instead are secreted into the urine. Ordinarily, as a small sugar molecule, mannitol is easily absorbed, but lactulose, as a larger molecule, is not. The ratio of these sugars in the urine is used to determine the health of the intestinal barrier and whether it is too leaky or is not allowing sufficient absorption.

Liver genomic testing. Liver detoxification is accomplished through the action of a family of detoxification enzymes that are heavily concentrated in liver cells but are found in all cells. The genes that determine the activity of the liver enzymes may have alterations that in turn affect their activity. These alterations are inherited and are referred to as genetic single nucleotide polymorphisms (SNPs). The presence of these SNPs can be measured by genetic analysis of blood cells. The presence or absence of these SNPs can help your doctor determine your detoxification capacity and susceptibilities.

Nutritional assessment. This is often desired by people with a history of cancer, particularly if they are making efforts to improve their diet. Simply measuring blood levels of nutrients is not always useful because the amount of a nutrient in the blood does not necessarily reflect the amount of that nutrient in body tissues where it is used. There are some nutritional tests that your doctor may order. These tests typically use whole blood cells to measure individual nutrients; for instance, magnesium can be accurately assessed from red blood cells. Another such test places a person's white blood cells into a test media that contains the minimal amount of nutrients required by the white blood cells to function. By sequentially removing and increasing each nutrient and measuring white blood cell activity, a determination can be made about the cell's nutrient status. With that, the body's level of that nutrient can be estimated. Although this test may indeed provide an indication of nutritional status, the results should be interpreted in the context of what is known about the person's diet, absorption, and medical history.

General Risk Assessment Testing

There are additional tests that provide a view into various areas of cancer risk that are not specifically tied to each of the five pathways.

Circulating tumor cells (CTCs). CTC tests capture cancer cells that are circulating in the blood. These cells can then be analyzed chemically and microscopically. This analysis can provide useful information about the nature of the cancer, identify potential targets for therapies, and may even give prognostic information. Some oncologists use these tests to help them learn about the molecular characteristics of an individual's cancer, which in turn helps determine their selection of therapies. These tests are still being studied, so they are not yet widely used. However, they offer a very promising way to learn about the state of an individual's cancer with a simple blood draw. CTCs are present in people with metastatic cancer and can be found in the blood of people with early-stage cancers. For instance, people who have received chemotherapy for early-stage breast cancer and who have CTCs after treatment have reduced survival rates. This is because circulating tumor cells have the potential to seed secondary tumors in other parts of the body. Knowing about the presence of CTCs after what is presumed to be definitive treatment creates the opportunity for additional (and different) treatment at a time when it really counts. The newer generation of the CTC test is much better at catching the tumor cells and also catching what appear to be microclusters of CTCs. These groupings of cancer cells may be directly implicated in metastasis.

Galectin-3. Galectin-3 molecule is normally present in small amounts throughout the body. An elevated level of galectin-3 is directly linked to inflammation and fibrosis and is now considered as a biomarker for risk of progression of cardiovascular disease. Cancerous cells express galectin-3 on their surfaces to help them stick onto the blood vessels so that they can move through the vessel and anchor themselves in sites distant from the original location of the tumor. Abnormally high levels of galectin-3 in the blood of people with cancer may be an indicator of the metastatic risk for that cancer. This test is available at standard reference labs, and clinical studies have correlated high galectin-3 levels with increased risk of cancers of the thyroid, kidney, and ovary as well as with increased risk of progressive disease in people already diagnosed with melanoma, lymphoma, and breast and colon cancer.

Telomeres. Telomeres are protective caps at the end of each chromosome that stabilize the DNA during cell division. As a cell ages, its telomeres become shorter. Eventually, the telomeres become too short to allow cell division. At this point, the cell undergoes apoptosis (cell suicide). This is a natural consequence of aging and is why we are not immortal beings. However, telomeres can become abnormally shortened in people exposed to oxidative insult, under significant stress, or as a result of chronic sleep deprivation, nutrient deficiencies, lack of exercise, and other lifestyle factors. Adults with prematurely shortened telomeres have unstable chromosomes and are at higher risk for the development of cancer. People already diagnosed with cancer who have shortened telomeres are at increased risk of dying from their cancer. A telomere test can determine the length of a patient's telomeres in relation to the patient's age. In this test, the patient's average telomere length in blood cells is compared to telomere lengths from a population sample in the same age range as the patient to determine the patient's percentile score and thereby gauge the sufficiency of telomere length.

Being Proactive

Achieving cancer-prevention success requires a shift in perspective. From the book *The Art of Possibility*, Rosamund Stone Zander and Benjamin Zander write: "Life often looks like an obstacle course. In order to maximize success, we spend a good

---

Thrive Thought

Tests and examinations are important components of a cancer-prevention plan. However, we need to keep all this testing in context of our desire to live a happy, fulfilling, and wonderful life. Seeking testing out of fear, especially when this testing only fuels our fear, is not productive to our health. Before obtaining any diagnostic or biomarker test, spend some time contemplating the value of the life that you are about to analyze—your life! As the poet Mary Oliver writes: "Tell me, what is it you plan to do with your one wild and precious life?" Armed with even a partial answer to that question will help you face tests, and their results, with greater peace and courage.

---

deal of time discussing what stands in the way of it." Let's not look at results from a screening test as a roadblock standing in the way of our happiness. Rather, let's look at it as information that will help us navigate the obstacle course of life. Partner with your doctor to determine what, if any, lab tests might be indicated and be prepared to use this information as street lamps illuminating your path to ongoing health and wellness. Keep your eye on the prize—thriving!

Simple Steps for Successful Screening

Embrace these simple steps as you think about proactive screening:

Know your body. Although proactive screening and regular checkups are a critical part of a cancer-prevention program, one of the best cancer-prevention strategies is to know your body. Pay attention to your body and the messages that your tissues are sending you every day. Get to know your muscle aches, places of weariness, appetite patterns, and energy levels. The more you know about you, the more likely that you will notice when something is amiss. Changes in how your body feels can be the first sign that something is not as it should be and that further medical evaluation is in order.

Create a health care team. The days of just having one health care practitioner are gone. We now have access to healing acupuncturists, massage therapists, naturopathic physicians, medical specialists, and many other people who can help us form our very own health care team. With your needs in mind, create a team that gives you comfort, safety, and support.

You are your best advocate. It's important to remember that you are in charge of your health care. Because of this, there are no silly questions, and there is no need to be intimidated by any member of your health care team. They are your allies, and you are your best advocate!

CHAPTER 7

Our Genes Are Not Our Destiny

We've covered a lot together—spirit, movement, diet, dietary supplements, and rejuvenation. Employing these five core strategies can positively and profoundly impact each of the body's five key pathways (the immune system, inflammation, hormonal balance, insulin resistance, and digestion and detoxification) to not only reduce your risk of developing cancer but also to live your life with vitality. In each of the areas of influence, we've given you critical action steps to help enhance that area of your life. Through this process, you will strengthen and transform your internal landscape to guard against a recurrence. And if you do get cancer again, you will be far better equipped to tackle it and move through it as a healthy person with cancer. We are often asked what makes the Five to Thrive Plan different. Of course, we feel there are many unique aspects, but one of the first things we like to bring up is that it is deeply rooted in science. Our plan is sandwiched in between bookends of scientific wisdom and logic, holding up to even the most meticulous scrutiny.

Strong Scientific Foundation

It is absolutely essential that the Five to Thrive Plan be built on a foundation of strong science. A risk reduction plan without scientific validation is like putting a big boulder on quicksand—it will soon disappear. We begin our scientific substantiation with the study of epigenetics. Simply put, epigenetics examines factors that influence the behavior of our genes. Our genes contain the instructions for who and what we are, but they do not function in a static manner. The ways in which they are expressed is influenced by their environment, our environment.

The foundation of epigenetics is the genome. Within each of our cells is a nucleus, which is home to our DNA. DNA is a coiled double helix that contains an individual's genome. The genome is estimated to contain twenty-five thousand to thirty thousand genes. Genes are made up of functional sequences of four different nucleotides. The order of the DNA nucleotides determines the message carried by that gene. This message is delivered in a process called transcription. Transcription occurs when an enzyme called RNA polymerase sweeps along unwound portions of the DNA, transcribing the genetic code. Each decoded message is contained in a unique strand of messenger RNA and used to make proteins, the ultimate workhorses of our cells. Proteins participate in cell repair, cell growth, energy production, toxin removal, and a host of other cellular activities.

Of course, what is read must be translated into action. Only the parts of the DNA that are unwound and exposed can be read. Here is where it gets interesting: the environment to which we expose ourselves through nutrition, environmental toxins, molecules of emotion, and other factors can dictate which parts of our DNA will be read. The environment of the cell influences which parts of our DNA remain tightly coiled and unreadable and which parts unwind to expose the genes in that segment to transcription. As the cellular environment changes, so too does our genetic expression. This dynamic silencing and activation of our genes is at the heart of epigenetics.

To understand the impact of epigenetics, think about identical twins. Identical twins share the exact same DNA, and when they are born, they are very difficult to tell apart. However, as twins age, differences become apparent. This is most dramatic when one twin develops a disease such as cancer, while the other remains healthy. If, for instance, one twin smoked cigarettes, which contain compounds that switch some genes on and others off, that twin's genome is epigenetically altered. In fact, cigarette smoke changes the behavior of dozens of genes, turning off key repair genes and turning on growth-promoter genes. Although the DNA in the twins is the same, the DNA's behavior is markedly different in the twin who smokes, putting that twin at risk of developing cancer, while the other twin has a greater chance of remaining cancer-free.

In a simplistic sense, cancer is ultimately the result of both normal expression of mutated genes or mutated expression of normal genes. In each case, factors external to the DNA are responsible for mutating the genes or their expression. External factors can also protect genes and promote healthy genetic expression. By altering these external factors through how we live our lives, we can transform our internal landscape and influence our genetic expression toward health and away from diseases such as cancer.

All of this is really cause for celebration. Our genes are not our destiny. We have the opportunity, through the choices we make, to change our genetic expression. Much like the musical notes on a page, the music that is *us* depends entirely upon how the notes are played. Although we cannot change our internal notes, we can play some loudly and others softly, and we can repeat some and skip others, changing the song completely. This is the beauty of the science of epigenetics, and it is at the core of the Five to Thrive Plan.

Healthy People Can Get Cancer

After most of our presentations on thriving after cancer, we take questions from the audience. We often receive a version of the same question: Why did I get cancer even though I had a great diet, I worked out, and I rarely got sick? One audience member in particular was very frustrated as she explained that she was only in her late thirties, had been a runner for years, was a vegetarian, and had no family history of cancer . . . and yet, she got cancer. Yes, a healthy person can still get cancer. Healthy people cannot exercise or eat away spontaneous DNA mutations from environmental exposures. Healthy people generally have healthy cells with stable DNA, but even then, cells can make simple, yet catastrophic, mistakes in DNA replication, cell repair, or cell division. Healthy people cannot change their inherited genes and, in some cases, cannot effectively compensate for these genetic susceptibilities through epigenetic alterations.

While this can be confusing, frustrating, and downright scary, it is important to remember that even though there is no ironclad prevention plan, we can significantly reduce our risk through healthful living. Healthy cells make for hardy DNA, which will provide increased resistance to cancer. Healthy people tend to continue to live healthy, vital lives despite having cancer. Their prognosis is often better, and they can often manage harsh treatments more effectively.

The bottom line is, if we do get cancer, it's best to be a *healthy* person with cancer!

For a Lifetime

We are fortunate. In every day there exist several moments that can become opportunities to thrive. There are moments to love, move, eat something healthy, take a supplement or two, and relax. When we string all of these moments together, we create a risk reduction plan that is no longer a plan; it's a way of living. We began *The Definitive Guide to Thriving After Cancer* with the concept of living a spirited life, and we will end the book in the same way. To live a spirited life is to infuse love, laugher, joy, service, and hope into your daily living. This not only gives life meaning, but it also brings meaning to your efforts, for a lifetime. Taking a dietary supplement is important, but if we are not feeling grateful, optimistic, and happy, the effect of that supplement will not be as powerful. We can eat a healthy diet or exercise three times a week, but if we find that to be drudgery, it will not likely be sustainable.

In every aspect of our lives, add a layer of spirit to each element of the Five to Thrive Plan. Spirit is the bond that holds the

Your Final Thrive Thought

Be gentle with yourself and those around you. Recognize that transformation takes time and thriving is a process, not a destination. Over time you will weave the concepts and philosophies of the Five to Thrive Plan into your daily life, your interactions with others, and your very being. But on those days or in those moments when you don't feel like a Thriver, remind yourself that the Thriver is there—always has been and always will be. Gently coax that Thriver out, and begin your journey anew.

As Henry David Thoreau wrote: "Thaw with her gentle persuasion is more powerful than Thor with his hammer. The one melts, the other breaks into pieces. The finest workers in stone are not copper or steel tools, but the gentle touches of air and water working at their leisure with a liberal allowance of time." And the great Vincent Van Gogh said: "Even the knowledge of my own fallibility cannot keep me from making mistakes. Only when I fall do I get up again." You are each, and all, remarkable individuals. You are important and matter deeply to this world. Treat yourself with gentle loving-kindness. Remember, it's always a good time to thrive!

entire plan together. It's the beginning, the middle, and the end. Spirit is what ensures the plan is sustainable. Most important, spirit is what makes the plan the most enjoyable! John F. Kennedy once reminded us that when the word "crisis" is written in Chinese, two letters are used. One letter represents danger and the other represents opportunity. As a Thriver, you have faced the danger. Now take advantage of the opportunity to heal from your crisis.

Dear Thriver, you can stand a little taller now and breathe a little easier. Remember, your journey through cancer has not ended; it is just beginning. You will never forget your cancer or its impact. But you have transcended your diagnosis and have moved into the realm of the Thriver. We encourage you to share your victory—and your wisdom—with others. As Thrivers, we have been given a gift, and that gift is meant to be shared.

Your Final Simple Steps to Living as a Thriver

We've come to our final recommendations in the book. We leave you with these two encouragements as you embark on your journey toward thriving.

Be a sponge. We have a unique opportunity to soak up as much knowledge, laughter, and joy this life has to give us. In every moment of every day we are given the perfect teacher, and that teacher is inside us, around us, and with us wherever we go.

Live in loving-kindness. We cannot say it better than inspired Buddhist teacher Pema Chodron: "When you begin to touch your heart or let your heart be touched, you begin to discover that it is bottomless, that it doesn't have any resolution, that this heart is huge, vast and limitless. You begin to discover how much warmth and gentleness there is, as well as how much space." Bathe yourself and those you love in kindness and compassion. Cultivate gratitude for the infinite blessings that we are presented with each day.

Resources

Following is a list of books, organizations, and websites that can provide additional valuable health information on a variety of topics. Please keep in mind that this is not meant to be an exhaustive list; however, the resources included here represent some of our favorites. Use them in your journey toward thriving!

Books

Inspirational

The Art of Possibility: Transforming Professional and Personal Life, by Rosamund Stone Zander and Benjamin Zander (Penguin, 2002)

The Book of Awakening: Having the Life You Want by Being Present to the Life You Have, by Mark Nepo (Conari, 2011)

The Chemistry of Calm: A Powerful, Drug-Free Plan to Quiet Your Fears and Overcome Your Anxiety, by Henry Emmons, MD (Touchstone, 2010)

The Chemistry of Joy: A Three-Step Program for Overcoming Depression through Western Science and Eastern Wisdom, by Henry Emmons, MD (Fireside, 2006)

The Introvert Advantage: How to Thrive in an Extrovert World, by Marti Olsen Laney (Workman, 2002)

Jungian 16 Types Personality Test: Find Your 4 Letter Archetype to Guide Your Work, Relationships, and Success, by Richard N. Stephenson (RichardStep.com Publishing, 2012)

Kitchen Table Wisdom: Stories That Heal, by Rachel Naomi Remen, MD (Riverhead, 2006)

My Grandfather's Blessings: Stories of Strength, Refuge, and Belonging, by Rachel Naomi Remen, MD (Riverhead, 2001)

The Power of Now: A Guide to Spiritual Enlightenment, by Eckhart Tolle (New World Library, 2004)

When Things Fall Apart: Heart Advice for Difficult Times, by Pema Chodron (Shambhala, 2000)

Why I Wake Early: New Poems, by Mary Oliver (Beacon, 2005)

Health

8 Weeks of Women's Wellness: The Detoxification Plan for Breast Cancer, Endometriosis, Infertility and Other Women's Health Conditions, by Marianne Marchese, ND (Smart Publications, 2011)

Chakra Foods for Optimum Health: A Guide to the Foods That Can Improve Your Energy, Inspire Creative Changes, Open Your Heart, and Heal Body, Mind, and Spirit, by Deanna Minnich, PhD, CN (Conari, 2009)

Definitive Guide to Cancer, 3rd Edition: An Integrative Approach to Prevention, Treatment, and Healing, by Lise Alschuler, ND, and Karolyn A. Gazella (Celestial Arts, 2010)

The Encyclopedia of Healing Foods, by Michael Murray, ND (Atria, 2005)

Fighting Cancer from Within: How to Use the Power of Your Mind for Healing, by Martin Rossman, MD (Holt, 2003)

Healing Depression, by Peter Bongiorno, ND, LAc (CCNM, 2010)

How to Talk with Your Doctor: The Guide for Patients and Their Physicians Who Want to Reconcile and Use the Best of Conventional and Alternative Medicine, by Ronald L. Hoffman, MD (Basic Health, 2006)

Life over Cancer: The Block Center Program for Integrative Cancer Treatment, by Keith Block, MD (Bantam, 2009)

One Bite at a Time: Nourishing Recipes for Cancer Survivors and Their Friends, by Rebecca Katz and Mat Edelson (Celestial Arts, 2008)

The Journey Through Cancer by Jeremy Geffen, MD (Three Rivers, 2006)

Sexy after Cancer, by Barbara Musser (SAC, 2012)

Sustainable Wellness: An Integrative Approach to Transform Your Mind, Body, and Spirit, by Matt Mumber, MD, and Heather Reed (New Page, 2012)

Unstuck: Your Guide to the Seven-Stage Journey out of Depression, by James S. Gordon, MD (Penguin, 2009)

What the Drug Companies Won't Tell You and Your Doctor Doesn't Know: The Alternative Treatments That May Change Your Life—and the Prescriptions That Could Harm You, by Michael Murray, ND (Atria, 2010)

Zest for Life: The Mediterranean Anti-Cancer Diet, by Conner Middelmann-Whitney (Honeybourne, 2011)

Fitness Assessment Tools

There are some excellent fitness assessment and tracking programs online, most of which are also available as apps for smartphones. These applications assists the user in creating and monitoring individualized diet and exercise plans based on their current weight, activity level, and fitness goals. Some of our favorites are:

- www.myfitnesspal.com
- www.sparkpeople.com
- www.fitday.com
- www.caloriecount.com

Organizations

American Academy of Environmental Medicine (www.aaemonline.org)

American Association of Naturopathic Physicians (www.naturopathic.org)

American Chiropractic Association (www.acatoday.org)

American College for Advancement in Medicine (www.acamnet.org)

American Holistic Medical Association (www.holisticmedicine.org)

National Center for Homeopathy (www.homeopathic.org)

Oncology Association of Naturopathic Physicians (www.oncanp.org)

Society for Integrative Oncology (www.integrativeonc.org)

Online Resources

4 Wholeness (www.4wholeness.com)

Annie Appleseed Project (www.annieappleseedproject.org)

Commonweal Health and Environmental Research Institute (www.commonweal.org)

Environmental Working Group (www.ewg.org)

Five to Thrive Plan (www.FivetoThrivePlan.com)

Healing Journeys (www.healingjourneys.org)

Karolyn A. Gazella (www.karolyngazella.com)

Lise Alschuler, ND, FABNO (www.drlise.net)

Natural Medicine Journal (www.naturalmedicinejournal.com)

Pink-Link (www.pink-link.org)

References by Chapter

Introduction: The Five to Thrive Plan

Alschuler, L., and K. Gazella. 2010. *The Definitive Guide to Cancer.* Third edition. New York: Random House.

Lally, P., C.H.M. van Jaarsveld, H.W.W. Potts, and J. Wardle. 2009. "How are habits formed: Modeling habit formation in the real world." *European Journal of Sociology* 40(6):998–1009.

Mariotto, A. B., et al. 2011. "Projections of the cost of cancer care in the United States: 2010–2020." *Journal of the National Cancer Institute* 103(2):117–28.

Niederdeppe, J., and A. G. Levy. 2007. "Fatalistic beliefs about cancer prevention and three prevention behaviors." *Cancer Epidemiology, Biomarkers, and Prevention* 16(5):998–1003.

Ornish, D., J. Lin, J. Daubenmier, G. Weidner, E. Epel, C. Kemp, M. J. Magbanua, R. Marlin, L. Yglecias, P. R. Carroll, and E. H. Blackburn. 2008. "Increased telomerase activity and comprehensive lifestyle changes: A pilot study." *Lancet Oncology* 9(11):1048–57.

Stull, A.J., K.C. Cash, W. D. Johnson, C.M. Champagne, and W.T. Cefalu. 2010. "Bioactives in blueberries improve insulin sensitivity in obese, insulin-resistant men and women." *Journal of Nutrition* 140(10):1764–8.

Zimmerman, G. L., C. G. Olsen, and M. F. Bosworth. 2000. "A 'stage of change' approach to helping patients change behavior." *American Family Physician* 61:1409–16.

Chapter 1. Enhance Your Spirit

Bränström, R., P. Kvillemo, and T. Akerstedt. 2012. "Effects of mindfulness training on levels of cortisol in cancer patients." *Psychosomatics* (December 3) S0033–3182(12).

Brown, Brené. 2010. "The Power of Vulnerability" (TED Talk, Houston, TX). www.ted.com/talks/brene_brown_on_vulnerability.html.

Christie, W., and C. Moore. 2005. "The impact of humor on patients with cancer." *Clinical Journal of Oncology Nursing* 9(2):211–18.

Costanzo, E. S., et al. 2005. "Psychosocial factors and interleukin-6 among women and advanced ovarian cancer." *Cancer* 104:305–13.

Dalmida, S. G., M. M. Holstad, C. Diiorio, and G. Laderman. 2009. "Spiritual well-being, depressive symptoms, and immune status among women living with HIV/AIDS." *Women's Health* 49(2–3):119–43.

Danner, D. D., D. A. Snowdon, and W. V. Friesen. 2001. "Positive emotions in early life and longevity: Finding from the nun study." *Journal of Personality and Social Psychology* 80(5):804–13.

DeMoor, J. S., et al. 2006. "Optimism, distress, health-related quality of life, and change in cancer antigen 125 among patients with ovarian cancer undergoing chemotherapy." *Psychosomatic Medicine* 68:555–62.

Emmons, R. A., and M.E. McCullough. 2003. "Counting blessings versus burdens: Experimental studies of gratitude and subjective well-being in daily life." *Journal of Personality and Social Psychology* 84:377–89.

Fuchs, C., et al. 2012. "Higher dietary glycemic load linked to worse colon cancer survival." *Journal of the National Cancer Institute* (November 7).

Hartley, T. A., S. S. Knox, D. Fekedulegn, et al. 2012. "Association between depressive symptoms and metabolic syndrome in police officers: Results from two cross-sectional studies." *Journal of the Environment and Public Health* (2012):861219–37.

Hayashi, T., and K. Murakami. 2009. "The effects of laughter on post-prandial glucose levels and gene expression in type 2 diabetic patients." *Life Science* (July 31) 85(5–6):185–87.

Hershberger, P. J. 2005. "Prescribing happiness: Positive psychology and family medicine." *Family Medicine* 37(9):630–34.

Holman, E. A., et al. 2008. "Terrorism, acute stress, and cardiovascular health: A 3-year national study following the September 11th attacks." *Archives of General Psychiatry* 65(1):73–80.

Li, X. J., Y. L. He, H. Ma, et al. 2012. "Prevalence of depressive and anxiety disorders in Chinese gastroenterological outpatients." *World Journal of Gastroenterology* 18(20):2561–68.

Marsland, A. L., S. D. Pressman, and S. Cohen. 2007. "Positive affect and immune function." In R. Ader, ed., *Psychoneuroimmunology*. 4th ed. Vol. 2. San Diego: Elsevier, 761–79.

McClelland, D., D. C. McClelland, and C. Kirchnit. 1988. "The effect of motivational arousal through films on salivary immunoglobulin A." *Psychology and Health* 2:31–52.

O'Donovan, A., et al. 2009. "Pessimism correlates with leukocyte telomere shortness and elevated interleukin-6 in post-menopausal women." *Brain, Behavior, and Immunity* 23(4):446–49.

Ong, A. D., D. K. Mroczek, and C. Riffin. 2011. "The health significance of positive emotions in adulthood and later life." *Social and Personality Psychology Compass* 5(8):538–51.

Pace, T. W., L. T. Negi, D. D. Adame, S. P. Cole, T. I. Sivilli, T. D. Brown, M. J. Issa, and C. L. Raison. 2009. "Effect of compassion meditation on neuroendocrine, innate immune, and behavioral responses to psychosocial stress." *Psychoneuroendocrinology* 34(1):87–98.

Phillips, A. C., et al. 2006. "Bereavement and marriage are associated with antibody response to influenza vaccination in the elderly." *Brain, Behavior, and Immunity* 20(3):279–89.

Ram, Dass. 1976. *Grist for the Mill*. Chicago, IL: Unity Press.

Rein, G., M. Atkinson, and R. McCraty. 1995. "The physiological and psychological effects of compassion and anger." *Journal of Advancements in Medicine* 8(2):87–105.

Schor, J. 2010. "Emotions and health: Laughter really is good medicine." *Natural Medicine Journal* 2(1).

Steptoe, A., K. O'Donnell, M. Marmot, and J. Wardle. 2008. "Positive affect, psychological well-being, and good sleep." *Journal of Psychosomatic Research* 64(4):409–15.

Steptoe, A., J. Wardle, and M. Marmot. 2005. "Positive affect and health-related neuroendocrine, cardiovascular, and inflamatory processes." *Proceedings of the National Academy of Sciences* 102:6508–12.

Watson, M., et al. 2005. "Influence of psychological response on breast cancer survival: 10-year follow-up of a population-based cohort." *European Journal of Cancer* 41(12):1710–14.

Zander, Rosamund, and Benjamin Zander. 2002. *The Art of Possibility: Transforming Professional and Personal Life.* New York: Penguin.

Zernicke, K. A., T. S. Campbell, P. K. Blustein, et al. 2012. "Mindfulness-based stress reduction for the treatment of irritable bowel syndrome symptoms: A randomized wait-list controlled trial." *International Journal of Behavioral Medicine* (May 23).

Chapter 2. Let's Move

Ağıl, A., F. Abike, A. Daşkapan, R. Alaca, and H. Tüzün. 2010. "Short-term exercise approaches on menopausal symptoms, psychological health, and quality of life in postmenopausal women." *Obstetrics and Gynecology International* [Epub August 16, 2010].

Arikawa, A. Y., W. Thomas, K. H. Schmitz, and M. S. Kurzer. 2011. "Sixteen weeks of exercise reduces C-reactive protein levels in young women." *Medicine and Science in Sports and Exercise* 43(6):1002–9.

Bilek, L., et al. 2012. "Exercise could fortify immune system against future cancers" (study presented at the Integrative Biology of Exercise VI meeting, Westminster, CO, October 10–13).

Bower, J. E., D. Garet, and B. Sternlieb. 2011. "Yoga for persistent fatigue in breast cancer survivors: Results of a pilot study." *Evidence-Based Complementary and Alternative Medicine* 1–8.

Chen X., W. Lu, Y. Zheng, K. Gu, Z. Chen, W. Zheng, and X. Shu. 2010. "Exercise, tea consumption, and depression among breast cancer survivors." *Journal of Clinical Oncology* 28:991–98.

Cohen, L., C. Warneke, R. T. Fouladi, M. A. Rodriguez, and A. Chaoul-Reich. 2004. "Psychological adjustment and sleep quality in a randomized trial of the effects of a Tibetan yoga intervention in patients with lymphoma." *Cancer* 100(10):2253–60.

Davies, N. J., L. Batehup, and R. Thomas. 2011. "The role of diet and physical activity in breast, colorectal, and prostate cancer survivorship: A review of the literature." *British Journal of Cancer* 105(S1):S52–S73.

Duclos, M., J. B. Corcuff, F. Pehourcq, and A. Tabarin. 2001. "Decreased pituitary sensitivity to glucocorticoids in endurance-trained men." *European Journal of Endocrinology* 144:363–68.

Dunstan, D., J. Shaw, B. Kingwell, et al. 2012. "Breaking up prolonged sitting reduces postprandial glucose and insulin responses." *Diabetes Care* 35(5):976–83.

Fairey, A.S., K. S. Courneya, C. J. Field, G. J. Bell, L. W. Jones, and J. R. Mackey. 2005. "Randomized controlled trial of exercise and blood immune function in postmenopausal breast cancer survivors." *Journal of Applied Physiology* 98(4):1534–40.

Friedenreich, C.M. 2011. "Physical activity and breast cancer: Review of the epidemiologic evidence and biologic mechanisms." *Recent Results in Cancer Research* 188:125–39.

Fuzhong, L., et al. 2012. "Tai Chi and postural stability in patients with Parkinson's disease." *New England Journal of Medicine* (February) 366:511–519.

Herring, M. P., et al. 2012. "Feasibility of exercise training for the short-term treatment of generalized anxiety disorder: A randomized controlled trial." *Psychotherapy and Psyhcosomatics* 81(1):21–28.

Holloway, W. D., and H. Joiner-Bey. 2002. *Water: The Foundation of Youth, Health, and Beauty*. Green Bay, WI: IMPAKT Health.

Irwin, M. L., A. McTiernan, J. E. Manson, C. A. Thomson, B. Sternfeld, M. L. Stefanick, J. Wactawski-Wende, L. Craft, D. Lane, L. W. Martin, and R. Chlebowski. 2011. "Physical activity and survival in postmenopausal women with breast cancer: Results from the Women's Health Initiative." *Cancer Prevention Research (Philadelphia)* 4(4):522–9.

Ivy, J. L. 1997. "Role of exercise training in the prevention and treatment of insulin resistance and non-insulin-dependent diabetes mellitus." *Sports Medicine* 24(5): 321–36.

Kenfield, S. A., M. J. Stampfer, E. Giovannucci, and J. M. Chan. 2011. "Physical activity and survival after prostate cancer diagnosis in the Health Professionals Follow-Up Study." *Journal of Clinical Oncology* 29(6):726–32.

Martins, R. A., M. T. Verissimo, M. J. Coelho e Silva, S. P. Cumming, and A. M. Teixeira. 2010. "Effects of aerobic and strength-based training on metabolic health indicators in older adults." *Lipids in Health and Disease* 9:76–82.

Musto, A., K. Jacobs, M. Nash, G. DelRossi, and A. Perry. 2010. "The effects of an incremental approach to 10,000 steps/day on metabolic syndrome components in sedentary overweight women." *Journal of Physical Activity and Health* 7(6):737–45.

Rikli, R. E., and C. J. Jones. 1999. "Development and validation of a functional fitness test for community-residing older adults." *Journal of Aging and Physical Activity* 7:129–61.

Rogers, C. J., L. H. Colbert, J. W. Greiner, S. N. Perkins, and S. D. Hursting. 2008. "Physical activity and cancer prevention: Pathways and targets for intervention." *Sports Medicine* 38(4):271–96.

Ryan, A. S. 2000. "Insulin resistance with aging: Effects of diet and exercise." *Sports Medicine* 30(5):327–46.

Stookey, J. D., F. Constant, B. M. Popkin, and C. D. Gardner. 2008. "Drinking water is associated with weight loss in overweight dieting women independent of diet and activity." *Obesity* 16(11):2481–88.

Taylor-Piliae, R. E., W. L. Haskell, N. A. Stotts, and E. S. Froelicher. 2006. "Improvement in balance, strength, and flexibility after 12 weeks of Tai Chi exercise in ethnic Chinese adults with cardiovascular disease risk factors." *Alternative Therapies in Health and Medicine* 12(2):50–58.

Thompson Coon, J., K. Boddy, K. Stein, R. Whear, J. Barton, and M. H. Depledge. 2011. "Does participating in physical activity in outdoor natural environments have a greater effect on physical and mental wellbeing than physical activity indoors?" *Environmental Science and Technology* 45(5):1761–72.

Vadiraja, H. S., M. R. Rao, R. Nagarathna, H. R. Nagendra, M. Rekha, N. Vanitha, K. S. Gopinath, B. S. Srinath, M. S. Vishweshwara, Y. S. Madhavi, B. S. Ajaikumar, S. R. Bilimagga, and N. Rao. 2009. "Effects of yoga program on quality of life and affect in early breast cancer patients undergoing adjuvant radiotherapy: A randomized controlled trial." *Complementary Therapies in Medicine* 17(5-6):274–80.

Wallberg-Henriksson, H., J. Rincon, and J. R. Zierath. 1998. "Exercise in the management of non–insulin-dependent diabetes mellitus." *Sports Medicine* 25(2):130.

Wiggins, M. S., and E. M. Simonavice. 2010. "Cancer prevention, aerobic capacity, and physical functioning in survivors related to physical activity: A recent review." *Cancer Management and Research* 92:157–64.

Chapter 3. Enrich Your Diet

Aggarwal, B., and S. Shishodia. 2006. "Molecular targets of dietary agents for prevention and therapy of cancer." *Biochemical Pharmacology* 71:1397–1421.

Aggarwal, B. B., M. E. Van Kuiken, X. H. Iyer, K. B. Harikumar, and B. Sung. 2009. "Molecular targets of nutraceuticals derived from dietary spices: Potential role in suppression of inflammation and tumorigenesis." *Experimental Biology and Medicine* 234(8):825–49.

Anand, P., A. Kunnumakara, C. Sundaram, K. Harikumar, et al. 2008. "Cancer is a preventable disease that requires major lifestyle changes." *Pharmaceutical Research* 25(9):2097 116.

Aune, D., D. Chan, D. Greenwood, et al. 2012. "Dietary fiber and breast cancer risk: A systemic review and meta-analysis of prospective studies." *Annals of Oncology* (January 10) 23(6):1394–402.

Beasley, J. M., P. A. Newcomb, A. Trentham-Dietz, J. M. Hampton, et al. 2011. "Post-diagnosis dietary factors and survival after invasive breast cancer." *Breast Cancer Research and Treatment* (January 1). [Epub ahead of print].

Betts, K. S. 2011. "Plastics and food sources: Dietary intervention to reduce BPA and DEHP." *Environmental Health Perspectives* (July) 119(7):A306.

Bhatia, E., C. Doddivenaka, X. Zhang, A. Bommareddy, et al. 2011. "Chemopreventive effects of dietary canola oil on colon cancer development." *Nutrition and Cancer* 63(2):242–47.

Brandt, K., et al. 2011. "Agroecosystem management and nutritional quality of plan foods: The case of organic fruits and vegetables." *Critical Reviews in Plant Sciences* 30(1):177–97.

Breneman, C. B., and L. Tucker. 2012. "Dietary fibre consumption and insulin resistance: The role of body fat and physical activity." *British Journal of Nutrition* 7:1–9.

Camargo, A., J. Ruano, J. M. Fernandez, L. D. Parnell, et al. 2010. "Gene expression changes in mononuclear cells in patients with metabolic syndrome after acute intake of phenol-rich virgin olive oil." *BMC Genomics.* (April 20) (11):253.

Castillo-Pichardo, L., M. M. Martínez-Montemayor, J. E. Martínez, K. M. Wall, L. A. Cubano, and S. Dharmawardhane. 2009. "Inhibition of mammary tumor growth and metastases to bone and liver by dietary grape polyphenols." *Clinical and Experimental Metastasis* 26(6):505–16.

Chen, S., S. R. Oh, S. Phung, G. Hur, J. J. Ye, S. L. Kwok, G. E. Shrode, M. Belury, L. S. Adams, and D. Williams. 2006. "Anti-aromatase activity of phytochemicals in white button mushrooms (*Agaricus bisporus*)." *Cancer Research* 66(24):12026–34.

Cohen, A. E., and C. S. Johnston. 2011. "Almond ingestion at mealtime reduces postprandial glycemia and chronic ingestion reduces hemoglobin A(1c) in individuals with well-controlled type 2 diabetes mellitus." *Metabolism* 60(9):1312–7.

Crinnion, W. J. 2010. "Organic foods contain higher levels of certain nutrients, lower levels of pesticides, and may provide health benefits for the consumer." *Alternative Medicine Review* 15(1):4–12.

Dong, J., J. Zou, and X. F. Yu. 2011. "Coffee drinking and pancreatic cancer risk: A meta-analysis of cohort studies." *World Journal of Gastroenterology* 17(9):1204–10.

Eliassen, A. H., S. J. Hendrickson, L. A. Brinton, et al. 2012. "Circulating carotenoids and risk of breast cancer: Pooled analysis of eight prospective studies." *Journal of the National Cancer Institute* 104(24):1905–16.

Ganesan, S., A. N. Faris, A. T. Comstock, Q. Wang, S. Nanua, M. B. Hershenson, and U. S. Sajjan. 2012. "Quercetin inhibits rhinovirus replication in vitro and in vivo." *Antiviral Research* 94(3):258–71.

Ghavipour, M., A. Saedisomeolia, M. Djalali, et al. 2012. "Tomato juice consumption reduces systemic inflammation in overweight and obese females." *British Journal of Nutrition* (October 15) 1–5.

Guha, N., M. Kwan, C. Quesenberry Jr., and E. Weltzien. 2009. "Soy isoflavones and risk of cancer recurrence in a cohort of breast cancer survivors: The Life After Cancer Epidemiology Study." *Breast Cancer Research and Treatment* 118(2):395–405.

Gunter, M., D. Hoover, H. Yu, S. Wassertheil-Smoller, et al. 2009. "Insulin, insulin-like growth factor-1, and risk of breast cancer in postmenopausal women." *Journal of the National Cancer Institute* 101:48–60.

Ho, V. W., K. Leung, A. Hsu, et al. 2011. "A low carbohydrate, high protein diet slows tumor growth and prevents cancer initiation." *Cancer Research* 71:4484–93.

Je, Y., and E. Giovannucci. 2012. "Coffee consumption and risk of endometrial cancer: Findings from a large up-to-date meta-analysis." *International Journal of Cancer* 131(7):1700–10.

Johnson, J. J. 2011. "Carnosol: A promising anti-cancer and anti-inflammatory agent." *Cancer Letters* 305(1):1–7.

Kado, K., A. Forsyth, P. R. Patel, and J. A. Schwartz. 2012. "Dietary supplements and natural products in breast cancer trials." *Frontiers in Bioscience* 4:546–67.

Karlsen, A., L. Retterstøl, P. Laake, I. Paur, et al. 2007. "Anthocyanins inhibit nuclear factor-kappaB activation in monocytes and reduce plasma concentrations of pro-inflammatory mediators in healthy adults." *Journal of Nutrition* 137(8):1951–54.

Kayashima, T., M. Mori, H. Yoshida, Y. Mizushina, and K. Matsubara. 2009. "1,4-Naphthoquinone is a potent inhibitor of human cancer cell growth and angiogenesis." *Cancer Letters* 278(1):34–40.

Li, G., D. Ma, Y. Zhang, W. Zheng, and P. Wang. 2012. "Coffee consumption and risk of colorectal cancer: A meta-analysis of observational studies." *Public Health Nutrition* 16(2):346–57.

Liu, R. H. 2004. "Potential synergy of phytochemicals in cancer prevention: Mechanism of action." *Journal of Nutrition* 134:3479S–3485S.

Marquart, L., L. Wiemer, J. Jones, and B. Jacob. 2003. "Whole grains health claims in the USA and other efforts to increase whole-grain consumption." *Proceedings of the Nutrition Society* 62:151–60.

Martin, K. 2006. "Targeting apoptosis with dietary bioactive agents." *Experimental Biology and Medicine* 231:117–29.

McAfee, A. J., E. M. McSorley, G. J. Cuskelly, A. M. Fearon, et al. 2011. "Red meat from animals offered a grass diet increases plasma and platelet n-3 PUFA in healthy consumers." *British Journal of Nutrition* 105(1):80–89.

McCullough, M., A. Patel, L. Kushi, R. Patel, et al. 2011. "Following cancer prevention guidelines reduces risk of cancer, cardiovascular disease and all-cause mortality." *Cancer Epidemiology, Biomarkers, and Prevention* (April 5) 20(6):1089–97.

Meadows, G. G. 2012. "Diet, nutrients, phtyochemicals, and cancer metastasis suppressor genes." *Cancer Metastasis Review* 31(3–4):331–454.

Meyerhardt, J. A., K. Sato, D. Niedzwiecki, et al. 2012. "Dietary glycemic load and cancer recurrence and survival in patients with stage III colon cancer: Findings from CALGB 89803." *Journal of the National Cancer Institute* 104(22):1702–11.

Nachman, K. E., G. Raber, K. A. Francesconi, A. Navas-Acien, and D. C. Love. 2012. "Arsenic species in poultry feather meal." *The Science of the Total Environment* 417–18:183–8.

Narod, S. A. 2011. "Alcohol and risk of breast cancer." *Journal of the American Medical Association* 306(17):1920–1.

Nechuta, S., X. O. Shu, H. L. Li, et al. 2012. "Prospective cohort study of tea consumption and risk of digestive system cancers: Results from the Shanghai Women's Health Study." *American Journal of Clinical Nutrition* 96(5):1056–63.

Nechuta, S. J., B. J. Caan, W. Y. Chen, W. Lu, Z. Chen, M. L. Kwan, S. W. Flatt, Y. Zheng, W. Zheng, J. P. Pierce, and X. O. Shu. 2012. "Soy food intake after diagnosis of breast cancer and survival: An in-depth analysis of combined evidence from cohort studies of US and Chinese women." *American Journal of Clinical Nutrition* 96(1):123–32.

Nova, E., O. Toro, P. Varela, I. López-Vidriero, G. Morandé, and A. Marcos. 2006. "Effects of a nutritional intervention with yogurt on lymphocyte subsets and cytokine production capacity in anorexia nervosa patients." *European Journal of Nutrition* 45(4):225–33.

Pérez-Jiménez, J., V. Neveu, F. Vos, and A. Scalbert. 2010. "Identification of the 100 richest dietary sources of polyphenols: An application of the Phenol-Explorer database." *European Journal of Clinical Nutrition* 64(S3):S112–S120.

Romagnolo, D., and O. Selmin. 2012. "Flavonoids and cancer prevention: A review of the evidence." *Journal of Nutrition in Gerontology and Geriatrics* 31:206–38.

Rosa, A., and H. Shizgal. 1984. "The Harris Benedict equation re-evaluated: Resting energy requirements and the body cell mass." *American Journal of Clinical Nutrition* 40:168–82.

Sang, L. X., B. Chang, X. H. Li, and M. Jiang. 2013. "Consumption of coffee associated with reduced risk of liver cancer: A meta-analysis." *BMC Gastroenterology* 13(1):34.

Schutze, M., H. Boeing, T. Pischon, J. Rehm, et al. 2011. "Alcohol attributable burden of incidence of cancer in eight European countries based on results from prospective cohort study." *British Medical Journal* 342:d1584.

Shafique, K., P. McLoone, K. Qureshi, H. Leung, C. Hart, and D. S. Morrison. 2012. "Coffee consumption and prostate cancer risk: Further evidence for inverse relationship." *Nutrition Journal* 11:42–56.

Shu, X. O., Y. Zheng, H. Cai, K. Gu, et al. 2009. "Soy food intake and breast cancer survival." *JAMA* 302(22):2437–43.

Smith-Spangler, C., et al. 2012. "Are organic foods safer or healthier than conventional alternatives?: A systemic review." *Annals of Internal Medicine* 157(5):348–66.

Spadafranca, A., C. Martinez Conesa, S. Sirini, and G. Testolin. 2010. "Effect of dark chocolate on plasma epicatechin levels, DNA resistance to oxidative stress and total antioxidant activity in healthy subjects." *British Journal of Nutrition* 103(7):1008–14.

Steck, S., et al. 2012. "Increased flavonoid intake reduced risk for aggressive prostate cancer" (study presented at the eleventh annual American Association of Cancer Research [AACR] International Conference on Frontiers in Cancer Prevention Research, Anaheim, CA, October 16–19).

Stull, A. J., K. C. Cash, W. D. Johnson, C. M. Champagne, W. T. Cefalu. 2010. "Bioactives in blueberries improve insulin sensitivity in obese, insulin-resistant men and women." *Journal of Nutrition* 140(10):1764–68.

van Dijk, S. J., E. J. Feskens, M. B. Bos, D. W. Hoelen, et al. 2009. "A saturated fatty acid-rich diet induces an obesity-linked proinflammatory gene expression profile in adipose tissue of subjects at risk of metabolic syndrome." *American Journal of Clinical Nutrition* 90(6):1656–64.

Villasenor, A., A. Ambs, R. Ballard-Barbash, K. Baumgartner, et al. 2011. "Dietary fiber is associated with circulating concentrations of C-reactive protein in breast cancer survivors: The HEAL study." *Breast Cancer Research and Treatment* 129(2):485–94.

Wang, Y., et al. 2012. "Coffee and tea consumption and risk of lung cancer: A dose-response analysis of observational studies." *Lung Cancer* 78(2):169–70.

Wendy, Y., B. R. Chen, S. E. Hankinson, G. A. Colditz, A. Colditz, and W. C. Willett. 2011. "Moderate alcohol consumption during adult life, drinking patterns, and breast cancer risk." *JAMA* 306(17):1884–90.

Yu, X., Z. Bao, J. Zou, and J. Dong. 2011. "Coffee consumption and risk of cancers: A meta-analysis of cohort studies." *BMC Cancer* 11:96.

Zick, S. M., D. K. Turgeon, S. K. Vareed, et al. 2011. "Phase II study of the effects of ginger root extract on eicosanoids in colon mucosa in people at normal risk for colorectal cancer." *Cancer Prevention and Research (Philadelphia)* 4(11):1929–37.

Chapter 4. Utilize Dietary Supplements

Ahonen, M. H., L. Tenkanen, L. Teppo, M. Hakama, and P. Tuohimaa. 2000. "Prostate cancer risk and prediagnostic serum 25-hydroxyvitamin D levels (Finland)." *Cancer Causes Control* 11(9):847–52.

Andreasen, A. S., N. Larsen, T. Pedersen-Skovsgaard, R. M. Berg, K. Møller, K. D. Svendsen, M. Jakobsen, and B. K. Pedersen. 2010. "Effects of *Lactobacillus acidophilus* NCFM on insulin sensitivity and the systemic inflammatory response in human subjects." *British Journal of Nutrition* 104(12):1831–38.

Antony, B., B. Merina, V. Iyer, N. Judy, et al. 2008. "A pilot cross-over study to evaluate human oral bioavailability of BCM-95 cg (biocurcumax), a novel bioenhanced preparation of curcumin." *Indian Journal of Pharmaceutical Sciences* 70(4):445–50.

Athar, M., J. H. Back, X. Tang, K. H. Kim, et al. 2007. "Resveratrol: A review of pre-clinical studies for human cancer prevention." *Applied Pharmacology* 224(3):274–83.

Bartoli, G. M., P. Palozza, G. Marra, F. Armelao, et al. 1993. "N-3 PUFA and alpha-tocopherol control of tumor cell proliferation." *Molecular Aspects of Medicine* 14(3):247–52.

Bettuzzi, S., M. Brausi, F. Rizzi, G. Castagnetti, et al. 2006. "Chemoprevention of human prostate cancer by oral administration of green tea catechins in volunteers with high-grade prostate intraepithelial neoplasia: A preliminary report from a one-year proof-of-principle study." *Cancer Research* 66(2):1234–40.

Black, H. S., and L. E. Rhodes. 2006. "The potential of omega-3 fatty acids in the prevention of non-melanoma skin cancer." *Cancer Detection and Prevention* 30(3):224–32.

Bocle, J.-C., and C. Thomann. 2005. "Effects of probiotics and prebiotics on flora and immunity in adults." *Agence Francaise de Securite Sanitaire des Aliments* (February):63–111.

Boge, T., M. Rémigy, S. Vaudaine, J. Tanguy, R. Bourdet-Sicard, and S. van der Werf. 2009. "A probiotic fermented dairy drink improves antibody response to influenza vaccination in the elderly in two randomised controlled trials." *Vaccine* 27(41):5677–84.

Boocock, D.J., G. E. Faust, K. R. Patel, et al. 2007. "Phase I dose escalation pharmacokinetic study in healthy volunteers of resveratrol, a potential cancer chemopreventive agent." *Cancer Epidemiology, Biomarkers, and Prevention* 16(6):1246–52.

Brown, V. A., K. R. Patel, M. Viskaduraki, J. A. Crowell, et al. 2010. "Repeat dose study of the cancer chemopreventive agent resveratrol in healthy volunteers: Safety, pharmacokinetics, and effect on the insulin-like growth factor axis." *Cancer Research* 70(22):9003–11.

Cani, P. D., and N. M. Delzenne. 2009. "Interplay between obesity and associated metabolic disorders: New insights into the gut microbiota." *Current Opinions in Pharmacology* 9:737–43.

Carpenter, D. O. 2008. "Environmental contaminants as risk factors for developing diabetes." *Reviews on Environmental Health* 23(1):59–74.

Chen, Y., and S. H. Tseng. 2007. "Review. Pro- and anti-angiogenesis effects of resveratrol." *In Vivo* 21(2):365–70.

Chen, Z., Q. Chen, H. Xia, and J. Lin. 2011. "Green tea drinking habits and esophageal cancer in southern China: A case-control study." *Asian Pacific Journal of Cancer Prevention* 12(1):229–33.

Cheng, A. L., C. H. Hsu, J. K. Lin, et al. 2001. "Phase I clinical trial of curcumin, a chemopreventive agent, in patients with high-risk or pre-malignant lesions." *Anticancer Research* 21:2895–00.

Chiu, A., J. L. Chan, D. G. Kern, S. Kohler, et al. 2005. "Double-blinded, placebo-controlled trial of green tea extracts in the clinical and histologic appearance of photoaging skin." *Dermatologic Surgery* 31:855–59.

Cruz-Correa, M., D. Shoskes, P. Sanches, et al. 2006. "Combination treatment with curcumin and quercetin of adenomas in familial adenomatous polyposis." *Clinical Gastroenterology and Hepatology* 4:1035–38.

Cuomo, J., G. Appendino, A. S. Dern, E. Schneider, et al. 2011. "Comparative absorption of a standardized curcuminoid mixture and its lecithin formulation." *Journal of Natural Products* 74(4):664–69.

de Vrese, M., P. Winkler, P. Rautenberg, T. Harder, et al. 2005. "Effect of *Lactobacillus gasseri* PA 16/8, *Bifidobacterium longum* SP 07/3, *B. bifidum* MF 20/5 on common cold episodes: A double blind, randomized, controlled trial." *Clinical Nutrition* 24(4):481–91.

Eastwood, G. L. 1996. "Pharmacologic prevention of colonic neoplasms. Effects of calcium, vitamins, omega fatty acids, and nonsteroidal anti-inflammatory drugs." *Digestive Diseases* 14(2):119–28.

Enyeart, J. A., H. Liu, J. J. Enyeart. 2009. "Curcumin inhibits ACTH- and angiotensin II-stimulated cortisol secretion and Ca(v)3.2 current." *Journal of Natural Products* 72(8):1533–37.

Fedirko, V., R. M. Bostick, W. D. Flanders, Q. Long, et al. 2009. "Effects of vitamin D and calcium supplementation on markers of apoptosis in normal colon mucosa: A randomized, double-blind, placebo-controlled clinical trial." *Cancer Prevention and Research* 2(3):213–23.

Fedirko, V., G. Torres-Mejía, D. Ortega-Olvera, C. Biessy, A. Angeles-Llerenas, E. Lazcano-Ponce, V. A. Saldaña-Quiroz, and I Romieu. 2012. "Serum 25-hydroxyvitamin D and risk of breast cancer: Results of a large population-based case-control study in Mexican women." *Cancer Causes Control* 23(7):1149–62.

Finocchiaro, C., O. Segre, M. Fadda, T. Monge, et al. 2012. "Effect of n-3 fatty acids on patients with advanced lung cancer: A double-blind, placebo-controlled study." *British Journal of Nutrition* 108(2):327–33.

Fotiadis, C., et al. 2008. "Role of probiotics, prebiotics, and synbiotics in chemoprevention for colorectal cancer." *World Journal of Gastroenterology* 14(42):6453–57.

Gago-Dominquez, M., E. Castelao, C.-L. Sun, D. Van Den Berg, et al. 2004. "Marine n-3 fatty acid intake, glutathione S-transferase polymorphisms and breast cancer risk in postmenopausal Chinese women in Singapore." *Carcinogenesis* 25(11):2143–47.

Gao, L., J. Wang, K. R. Sekhar, H. Yin, et al. 2007. "Novel n-3 fatty acid oxidation products activate Nrf2 by destabilizing the association between Keap1 and Cullin3." *Journal of Biological Chemistry* 282(4):2529–37.

Gao, Y. T., J. K. McLaughlin, W. J. Blot, B. T. Ji, et al. 1994. "Reduced risk of esophageal cancer associated with green tea consumption." *Journal of the National Cancer Institute* 86(11):855 58.

Garland, C., W. Grant, S. Mohr, et al. 2007. "What is the dose-response relationship between vitamin D and cancer risk?" *Nutrition Reviews* 65(8):S91–S95.

Gifkins, D., S. H. Olson, K. Demissie, S. E. Lu, A. N. Kong, and E. V. Bandera. 2012. "Total and individual antioxidant intake and endometrial cancer risk: Results from a population-based case-control study in New Jersey." *Cancer Causes Control* 23(6):887–95.

Golombick, T., T. H. Diamond, A. Manoharan, and R. Ramakrishna. 2012. "Monoclonal gammopathy of undetermined significance, smoldering multiple myeloma, and curcumin: A randomized, double-blind placebo-controlled cross-over 4g study and an open-label 8g extension study." *American Journal of Hematology* 87(5):455–60.

Goodwin, P. J., M. Ennis, K. I. Pritchard, J. Koo, and N. Hood. 2009. "Prognostic effects of 25-hydroxy vitamin D levels in early breast cancer." *Journal of Clinical Oncology* (May 18) 27(23):2757–63.

Gorham, E. D., C. F. Garland, F. C. Garland, W. B. Grant, et al. 2007. "Optimal vitamin D status for colorectal cancer prevention: A quantitative meta analysis." *American Journal of Preventive Medicine* 32(3):210–16.

Greenlee, H., M. L. Kwan, L. H. Kushi, J. Song, A. Castillo, E. Weltzien, C. P. Quesenberry Jr., and B. J. Caan. 2012. "Antioxidant supplement use after breast cancer diagnosis and mortality in the Life After Cancer Epidemiology (LACE) cohort." *Cancer* 118(8):2048–58.

Gupta, S., T. K. Sharma, G. G. Kaushik, and V. P. Shekhawat. 2011. "Vitamin E supplementation may ameliorate oxidative stress in type 1 diabetes mellitus patients." *Clincal Laboratory* 57(5–6):379–86.

Heller, A. R., T. Rössel, B. Gottschlich, O. Tiebel, et al. 2004. "Omega-3 fatty acids improve liver and pancreas function in postoperative cancer patients." *International Journal of Cancer* 111(4):611–16.

Holub, B., L. J. Hoffer, and P. Jones. 2002. "Clinical nutrition: Omega-3 fatty acids in cardiovascular care." *Canadian Medical Association Journal* 166(5):608–15.

Howells, L. M., D. P. Berry, P. J. Elliott, E. W. Jacobson, E. Hoffmann, B. Hegarty, K. Brown, W. P. Steward, and A. J. Gescher. 2011. "Phase I randomized, double-blind pilot study of micronized resveratrol (SRT501) in patients with hepatic metastases—safety, pharmacokinetics, and pharmacodynamics." *Cancer Prevention and Research (Philadelphia)* 4(9):1419–25.

Inoue, M., K. Tajima, M. Mizutani, H. Iwata, et al. 2001. "Regular consumption of green tea and the risk of breast cancer recurrence: Follow-up study from the Hospital-based Epidemiologic Research Program at Aichi Cancer Center (HERPACC), Japan." *Cancer Letters* 167(2):175–82.

Ishikawa, H., I. Akedo, T. Otani, T. Suzuki, et al. 2005. "Randomized trial of dietary fiber and *Lactobacillus casei* administration for prevention of colorectal tumors." *International Journal of Cancer* 116(5):762–67.

Iwasaki, M., M. Inoue, S. Sasazuki, et al. 2010. "Green tea drinking and subsequent risk of breast cancer in a population-based cohort of Japanese women." *Breast Cancer Research* 12:R88.

Jazayeri, S., S. A. Keshavarz, M. Tehrani-Doost, M. Djalali, M. Hosseini, H. Amini, M. Chamari, and A. Djazayery. 2010. "Effects of eicosapentaenoic acid and fluoxetine on plasma cortisol, serum interleukin-1 beta and interleukin-6 concentrations in patients with major depressive disorder." *Psychiatry Research* 178(1):112–15.

Joe, A. K., H. Liu, M. Suzui, M. E. Vural, D. Xiao, and I. B. Weinstein. 2002. "Resveratrol induces growth inhibition, S-phase arrest, apoptosis, and changes in biomarker expression in several human cancer cell lines." *Clinical Cancer Research* 8(3):893–903.

John, E. M., J. Koo, and G. G. Schwartz. 2007. "Sun exposure and prostate cancer risk: Evidence for a protective effect of early-life exposure." *Cancer Epidemiology, Biomarkers, and Prevention* 16(6):1283–86.

Kajander, K., E. Myllyluoma, M. Rajilić-Stojanović, S. Kyrönpalo, et al. 2008. "Clinical trial: Multispecies probiotic supplementation alleviates the symptoms of irritable bowel syndrome and stabilizes intestinal microbiota." *Alimentary Pharmacology and Therapeutics* 27(1):48–57.

Kumar, M., A. Kumar, R. Nagpal, D. Mohania, et al. 2010. "Cancer-preventing attributes of probiotics: An update." *International Journal of Food Science and Nutrition* 61(5):473–96.

Kunnumakkara, A., S. Guha, and B. Aggarwal. 2009. "Curcumin and Colorectal Cancer: Add Spice to Your Life." *Current Colorectal Cancer Reports* 5:5–14.

la Porte, C., N. Voduc, G. Zhang, I. Seguin, et al. 2010. "Steady-state pharmacokinetics and tolerability of trans-resveratrol 2000 mg twice daily with food, quercetin, and alcohol (ethanol) in healthy human subjects." *Clinical Pharmacokinetics* 49(7):449–54.

Lappe, J. M., D. Travers-Gustafson, K. M. Davies, R. R. Recker, and R. P. Heaney. 2007. "Vitamin D and calcium supplementation reduces cancer risk: Results of a randomized trial." *American Journal of Clinical Nutrition* 85:1586–91.

Li, Y.-H., Y. Wu, H. C. Wei, Y.Y. Xu, et al. 2009. "Protective effects of green tea extracts on photoaging and photoimmunosuppression." *Skin Research Technology* 15:338–45.

Liu, J., J. Xing, and Y. Fei. 2008. "Green tea (*Camellia sinensis*) and cancer prevention: A systematic review of randomized trials and epidemiological studies." *Chinese Medicine* 3:12.

Liu, Z. H., M. J. Huang, X. W. Zhang, L. Wang, et al. 2012. "The effects of perioperative probiotic treatment on serum zonulin concentration and subsequent postoperative infectious complications after colorectal cancer surgery: A double-center and double-blind randomized clinical trial." *American Journal of Clinical Nutrition* (December 12) 97(1):117–26.

Lopez-Huertas, E. 2012. "The effect of EPA and DHA on metabolic syndrome patients: A systematic review of randomised controlled trials." *British Journal of Nutrition* 107(Suppl 2):S185–94.

Mawer, E., J. Walls, A. Howell, et al. 1997. "Serum 1,25-dihydroxy vitamin D may be related inversely to disease activity in breast cancer patients with bone metastases." *Journal of Clinical Endocrinology and Metabolism* 82:118–22.

Mebarek, S., N. Ermak, A. Benzaria, S. Vicca, M. Dubois, G. Némoz, M. Laville, B. Lacour, E. Véricel, M. Lagarde, and A. F. Prigent. 2009. "Effects of increasing docosahexaenoic acid intake in human healthy volunteers on lymphocyte activation and monocyte apoptosis." *British Journal of Nutrition* 101(6):852–58.

Messaoudi, M., R. Lalonde, N. Violle, H. Javelot, D. Desor, A. Nejdi, J. F. Bisson, C. Rougeot, M. Pichelin, M. Cazaubiel, and J.M. Cazaubiel. 2011. "Assessment of psychotropic-like properties of a probiotic formulation (*Lactobacillus helveticus* R0052 and *Bifidobacterium longum* R0175) in rats and human subjects." *British Journal of Nutrition* 105:755–64.

Mikelsaar, M., J. Stsepetova, P. Hütt, H. Kolk, E. Sepp, K. Lõivukene, K. Zilmer, and M. Zilmer. 2010. "Intestinal *Lactobacillus* sp. is associated with some cellular and metabolic characteristics of blood in elderly people." *Anaerobe* 16:240–46.

Murff, H. J., M. J. Shrubsole, Q. Cai, W. E. Smalley, Q. Dai, G. L. Milne, R. M. Ness, and W. Zheng. 2012. "Dietary intake of PUFAs and colorectal polyp risk." *American Journal of Clinical Nutrition* 95(3):703–12.

Murphy, R. A., M. Mourtzakis, Q. S. Chu, V. E. Baracos, T. Reiman, and V. C. Mazurak. 2011. "Supplementation with fish oil increases first-line chemotherapy efficacy in patients with advanced nonsmall cell lung cancer." *Cancer* 117(16):3774–80.

Nakachi, K., K. Suemasu, K. Suga, T. Takeo, K. Imai, and Y. Higashi. 1998. "Influence of drinking green tea on breast cancer malignancy among Japanese patients." *Japanese Journal of Cancer Research* 89(3):254–61.

Nantz, M., C. A. Rowe, J. F. Bukowski, and S. S. Percival. 2009. "Standardized capsule of *Camellia sinensis* lowers cardiovascular risk factors in a randomized, double-blind, placebo-controlled study." *Nutrition* 25:147–54.

Narayanan, B. A., N. K. Narayanan, G. G. Re, and D. W. Nixon. 2003. "Differential expression of genes induced by resveratrol in LNCaP cells: P53-mediated molecular targets." *International Journal of Cancer* 104(2):204–12.

National Health and Nutrition Examination Survey. "What we eat in America, 2005–2006." Online at www.ars.usda.gov/ba/bhnrc/fsrg.

Norrish, A. E., C. M. Skeaff, G. L. Arribas, S. J. Sharpe, and R. T. Jackson. 1999. "Prostate cancer risk and consumption of fish oils: A dietary biomarker-based case-control study." *British Journal of Cancer* 81(7):1238–42.

Obi, Y., N. Ichimaru, T. Hamano, K. Tomida, et al. 2012. "Orally active vitamin D for potential chemoprevention of posttransplant malignancy." *Cancer Prevention and Research (Philadelphia)* 5(10):1229–35.

Ouwehand, A. C., N. Bergsma, R. Parhiala, S. Lahtinen, et al. 2008. "*Bifidobacterium microbiota* and parameters of immune function in elderly subjects." *FEMS Immunology and Medical Microbiology* 53(1):18 25.

Patel, K. R., V. A. Brown, D. J. Jones, R. G. Britton, et al. 2010. "Clinical pharmacology of resveratrol and its metabolites in colorectal cancer patients." *Cancer Research* 70(19):7392–99.

Peters, E. M., R. Anderson, D. C. Nieman, H. Fickl, and V. Jogessar. 2001. "Vitamin C supplementation attenuates the increases in circulating cortisol, adrenaline and anti-inflammatory polypeptides following ultramarathon running." *International Journal of Sports Medicine* 22(7):537–43.

Protiva, P., H.S. Cross, M.E. Hopkins, E. Kállay, G. Bises, E. Dreyhaupt, L. Augenlicht, M. Lipkin, M. Lesser, E. Livote, and P.R. Holt. 2009. "Chemoprevention of colorectal neoplasia by estrogen: Potential role of vitamin D activity." *Cancer Prevention Research (Philadelphia)* 2(1):43–51.

Prucksunand, C., B. Indrasukhsri, M. Leethochawalit, and K. Hungspreugs. 2001. "Phase II clinical trial on effect of the long turmeric (*Curcuma longa* Linn) on healing of peptic ulcer." *Southeast Asian Journal of Tropical Medicine and Public Health* 32:208–15.

Puertollano, M. A., E. Puertollano, G. A. de Cienfuegos, and M. A. de Pablo. 2011. "Dietary antioxidants: Immunity and host defense." *Current Topics in Medicinal Chemistry* (April 21) 11(14):1752–66.

Rafter, J., M. Bennett, G. Caderni, Y. Clune, et al. 2007. "Dietary synbiotics reduce cancer risk factors in polypectomized and colon cancer patients." *American Journal of Clinical Nutrition* 85:488–96.

Reale, M., P. Boscolo, V. Bellante, C. Tarantelli, M. Di Nicola, L. Forcella, Q. Li, K. Morimoto, and R. Muraro. 2012. "Daily intake of *Lactobacillus casei* Shirota increases natural killer cell activity in smokers." *British Journal of Nutrition* 108(2):308–14.

Rifatbegovic, Z., D. Mesic, F. Ljuca, M. Zildzic, M. Avdagic, K. Grbic, M. Agic, and B. Hadziefendic. 2010. "Effect of probiotics on liver function after surgery resection for malignancy in the liver cirrhotic." *Medical Archives* 64(4):208–11.

Ringel-Kulka, T., O. S. Palsson, D. Maier, I. Carroll, J. A. Galanko, G. Leyer, and Y. Ringel. 2011. "Probiotic bacteria *Lactobacillus acidophilus* NCFM and *Bifidobacterium lactis* Bi-07 versus placebo for the symptoms of bloating in patients with functional bowel disorders: A double-blind study." *Journal of Clinical Gastroenterology* 45(6):518–25.

Rosen, C. 2011. "Vitamin D insufficiency." *New England Journal of Medicine* 364:248–54.

Saggar, J. K., J. Chen, P. Corey, and L. U. Thompson. 2010. "Dietary flaxseed lignan or oil combined with tamoxifen treatment affects MCF-7 tumor growth through estrogen receptor- and growth factor-signaling pathways." *Molecular Nutrition and Food Research* 54(3):415–25.

Setiawan, V. W., Z. F. Zhang, G. P. Yu, Q. Y. Lu, et al. 2001. "Protective effect of green tea on the risks of chronic gastritis and stomach cancer." *International Journal of Cancer* 92(4):600–4.

Shanafelt, T. D., T. G. Call, C. S. Zent, J. F. Leis, et al. 2013. "Phase 2 trial of daily, oral polyphenon E in patients with asymptomatic, Rai stage 0 to II chronic lymphocytic leukemia." *Cancer* 119(2):363–70.

Shimizu, M., Y. Fukutomi, M. Ninomiya, K. Nagura, et al. 2008. "Green tea extracts for the prevention of metachronous colorectal adenomas: A pilot study." *Cancer Epidemiology, Biomarkers, and Prevention* 17(11):3020–5.

Showell, M. G., J. Brown, A. Yazdani, M. T. Stankiewicz, and R. J. Hart. 2011. "Antioxidants for male subfertility." *Cochrane Database of Systematic Reviews* (January 19) (1):CD007411.

Sijben, J. W., and P. C. Calder. 2007. "Differential immunomodulation with long-chain n-3 PUFA in health and chronic disease." *Proceedings of the Nutrition Society* 66(2):237–59.

Silva Jde, A., E. B. Trindade, M. E. Fabre, V. M. Menegotto, S. Gevaerd, S. Buss Zda, and T. S. Frode. 2012. "Fish oil supplement alters markers of inflammatory and nutritional status in colorectal cancer patients." *Cancer* 64(2):267–73.

Viljanen, M., M. Kuitunen, T. Haahtela, K. Juntunen-Backman, R. Korpela, and E. Savilahti. 2005. "Probiotic effects on faecal inflammatory markers and on faecal IgA in food allergic atopic eczema/dermatitis syndrome infants." *Pediatric Allergy and Immunology* 16:65–71.

Walle, T., F. Hsieh, M. H. DeLegge, J. E. Oatis Jr., and U. K. Walle. 2004. "High absorption but very low bioavailability of oral resveratrol in humans." *Drug Metabolism and Disposition* 32(12):1377–82.

West, N. J., S. K. Clark, R. K. Phillips, J. M. Hutchinson, R. J. Leicester, A. Belluzzi, and M. A. Hull. 2010. "Eicosapentaenoic acid reduces rec tal polyp number and size in familial adenomatous polyposis." *Gut* 59(7):918–25.

Willemsen, L. E., M. A. Koetsier, M. Balvers, C. Beermann, B. Stahl, and E. A. van Tol. 2008. "Polyunsaturated fatty acids support epithelial barrier integrity and reduce IL-4 mediated permeability in vitro." *European Journal of Nutrition* 47(4):183–91.

Wu, M., K. A. Harvey, N. Ruzmetov, Z. R. Welch, et al. 2005. "Omega-3 polyunsaturated fatty acids attenuate breast cancer growth through activa- tion of a neutral sphingomyelinase-mediated pathway." *International Journal of Cancer* 117(3):340–48.

Yuan, J. M., C. Sun, and L. M. Butler. 2011. "Tea and cancer prevention: Epidemiological studies." *Pharmacology Research* 64(2):123–35.

Zeng, J., Y. Q. Li, X. L. Zuo, Y. B. Zhen, J. Yang, and C. H. Liu. 2008. "Clini- cal trial: Effect of active lactic acid bacteria on mucosal barrier function in patients with diarrhoea-predominant irritable bowel syndrome." *Alimentary Pharmacology and Therapeutics* 28(8):994–1002.

Zhu, W., W. Qin, K. Zhang, G. E. Rottinghaus, Y. C. Chen, B. Kliethermes, and E. R. Sauter. 2012. "Trans-resveratrol alters mammary promoter hypermethylation in women at increased risk for breast cancer." *Nutrition and Cancer* 64(3):393–400.

Zou, J., J. Dong, and X. Yu. 2009. "Meta-analysis: *Lactobacillus* containing quadruple therapy versus standard triple first-line therapy for *Helicobacter pylori* eradication." *Helicobacter* 14(5):97–107.

Chapter 5. Create Rejuvenation

Baikie, K. A., and K. Wilhelm. 2005. "Emotional and physical health benefits of expressive writing." *Advances in Psychiatric Treatment* 11:338–46.

Bertini, G., V. Colavito, C. Tognoli, P. F. Etet, and M. Bentivoglio. 2010. "The aging brain, neuroinflammatory signaling and sleep-wake regulation." *Italian Journal of Anatomy and Embryology* 115(1–2):31–38.

Dibner, C., U. Schibler, and U. Albrecht. 2010. "The mammalian circadian timing system: Organization and coordination of central and peripheral clocks." *Annual Review of Physiology* 72.517–49.

Donga, E., M. van Dijk, J. G. van Dijk, N. R. Biermasz, G. J. Lammers, K. W. van Kralingen, E. P. Corssmit, and J. A. Romijn. 2010. "A single night of partial sleep deprivation induces insulin resistance in multiple metabolic pathways in healthy subjects." *Journal of Clinical Endocrinology and Metabolism* 95(6):2963–68.

Duez, H., and B. Staels. 2009. "Rev-erb-alpha: An integrator of circadian rhythms and metabolism." *Journal of Applied Physiology* 107(6):1972–80.

Faraut, B., K. Z. Boudjeltia, M. Dyzma, A. Rousseau, E. David, P. Stenuit, T. Franck, P. Van Antwerpen, M. Vanhaeverbeek, and M. Kerkhofs. 2011. "Benefits of napping and an extended duration of recovery sleep on alertness and immune cells after acute sleep restriction." *Brain, Behavior, and Immunity* 25(1):16–24.

Hansen, J., and C. Lassen. 2012. "Nested case-control study of night shift work and breast cancer risk among women in the Danish military." *Occupational and Environmental Medicine* (May) 69(8):551–6.

Irwin, M. 2002. "Effects of sleep and sleep loss on immunity and cytokines." *Brain, Behavior, and Immunity* 16(5):503–12.

Kang, D. H., T. McArdle, N. J. Park, M. T. Weaver, and B. Smith. 2011. "Dose effects of relaxation practice on immune responses in women newly diagnosed with breast cancer: An exploratory study." *Journal of Oncology Nursing Forum* 38(3):E240–52.

Kripke, D. F., R. D. Langer, and L. E. Kline. 2012. "Hypnotics' association with mortality or cancer: A matched cohort study." *British Medical Journal Open* 2(1):e000850.

Kryger, M. H., E. Mignot, W. C. Orr, D. Ryan, and J. K. Walsh. 2002. National Sleep Foundation. Sleep in America Poll.

Mullington, J. M., N. S. Simpson, H. K. Meier-Ewert, and M. Haack. 2010. "Sleep loss and inflammation." *Best Practice and Research Clinical Endocrinology and Metabolism* 24(5):775–84.

Nosek, M., H. P. Kennedy, Y. Beyene, D. Taylor, C. Gilliss, and K. Lee. 2010. "The effects of perceived stress and attitudes toward menopause and aging on symptoms of menopause." *Journal of Midwifery and Women's Health* 55(4):328–34.

Parent, M. É., M. El-Zein, M. C. Rousseau, J. Pintos, and J. Siemiatycki. 2012. "Night work and the risk of cancer among men." *American Journal of Epidemiology* 176(9):751–59.

Rafalson, L., R. P. Donahue, S. Stranges, M. J. Lamonte, J. Dmochowski, J. Dorn, and M. Trevisan. 2010. "Short sleep duration is associated with the development of impaired fasting glucose: The Western New York Health Study." *Annals of Epidemiology* 20(12):883–89.

Shurlygina, A. V., S. V. Mitshurina, L. V. Verbitskaja, A. Belkin, et al. 2010. "Structure of nuclear chromatin in cells of lymphoid organs and blood from mice maintained under abnormal light-dark cycle and treated with benz(a)pyrene." *Bulletin of Experimental Biology and Medicine* 149(1):29–32.

Stuckey, H. L., and J. Nobel. 2010. "The connection between art, healing, and public health: A review of current literature." *American Journal of Public Health* 100(2):254–63.

Wynn, E., M. A. Krieg, J. M. Aeschlimann, and P. Burckhardt. 2009. "Alkaline mineral water lowers bone resorption even in calcium sufficiency: Alkaline mineral water and bone metabolism." *Bone* 44(1):120–24.

Wynn, E., M. A. Krieg, S. A. Lanham-New, and P. Burckhardt. 2010. "Post-graduate Symposium: Positive influence of nutritional alkalinity on bone health." *Proceedings of the Nutrition Society* 69(1):166–73.

Zaharna, M., and C. Guilleminault. 2010. "Sleep, noise, and health: Review." *Noise Health* 12(47):64–69.

Chapter 6. Screening Strategies That Make Sense

Andrew, M. D., et al. 2010. "American Cancer Society guidelines for early detection of prostate cancer: Update." *CA: A Cancer Journal for Clinicians* 60:70–98.

Barrow, H., J. M. Rhodes, and L. G. Yu. 2012. "Simultaneous determination of serum galectin-3 and -4 levels detects metastases in colorectal cancer patients." *Cellular Oncology (Dordrecht)* (November 2) 36(1):9–13.

Bisset, L. R., T. L. Lung, M. Kaelin, E. Ludwig, and R. W. Dubs. 2004. "Reference values for peripheral blood lymphocyte phenotypes applicable to the healthy adult population in Switzerland." *European Journal of Haematology* 72(3):203–12.

Braeuer, R. R., M. Zigler, T. Kamiya, A. S. Dobroff, L. Huang, W. Choi, D. J. McConkey, E. Shoshan, A. K. Mobley, R. Song, A. Raz, and M. Bar-Eli. 2012. "Galectin-3 contributes to melanoma growth and metastasis via regulation of NFAT1 and Autotaxin." *Cancer Research* 72(22):5757–66.

Cunningham, D., et al. 2010. "Colorectal cancer." *Lancet* 375:1030–47.

Drazer, M. W., et al. 2011. "Population-based patterns and predictors of prostate-specific antigen screening among older men in the United States." *Journal of Clinical Oncology* 29(13):1763–43.

Eiró, N., L. González, L. O. González, B. Fernandez-Garcia, M. L. Lamelas, L. Marín, S. González-Reyes, J. M. Del Casar, and F. J. Vizoso. 2012. "Relationship between the inflammatory molecular profile of breast carcinomas and distant metastasis development." *PLoS One* 7(11).

Elit, L., et al. 2010. "Follow-up for women after treatment for cervical cancer." *Current Oncology* 17(3):65–69.

Fuhrman, B. J., C. Schairer, M. H. Gail, J. Boyd-Morin, X. Xu, L.Y. Sue, S. S. Buys, C. Isaacs, L. K. Keefer, T. D.Veenstra, C. D. Berg, R. N. Hoover, and Z. G. Ziegler. 2012. "Estrogen metabolism and risk of breast cancer in postmenopausal women." *Journal of the National Cancer Institute* 104(4):326–39.

Gallo,V., G. Leonardi, B. Genser, M. J. Lopez-Espinosa, S. J. Frisbee, L. Karlsson, A. M. Ducatman, and T. Fletcher 2012. "Serum perfluorooctanoate (PFOA) and perfluorooctane sulfonate (PFOS) concentrations and liver function biomarkers in a population with elevated PFOA exposure." *Environmental Health Perspectives* 120(5):655–60.

Kulie, T., et al. 2011. "Obesity and women's health: An evidence-based review." *Journal of the American Board of Family Medicine* 24:75–85.

Kurman, R. J., et al. 2008. "Early detection and treatment of ovarian cancer: Shifting from early stage to minimal volume of disease based on a new model of carcinogenesis." *American Journal of Obstetrics and Gynecology* 198(4):351–56.

Lin, J., I. M. Lee,Y. Song, N. R. Cook, J. Selhub, J. E. Manson, J. E. Buring, and S. M. Zhang. 2010. "Plasma homocysteine and cysteine and risk of breast cancer in women." *Cancer Research* 70(6):2397–405.

Matesa-Anić, D., S. Moslavac, N. Matesa, H. Cupić, and Z. Kusić. 2012. "Intensity and distribution of immunohistochemical expression of galectin-3 in thyroid neoplasms." *Acta Clinica Croatica* 51(2):237–41.

Melvin, J. C., C. Rodrigues, L. Holmberg, H. Garmo, N. Hammar, I. Jungner, G.Walldius, M. Lambe,W. Jassem, and M.Van Hemelrijck. 2012. "Gamma-glutamyl transferase and C-reactive protein as alternative markers of metabolic abnormalities and their associated comorbidites: A prospective cohort study." *International Journal of Molecular Epidemiology and Genetics* 3(4):276–85.

Mishra, A., and G. K. Makharia. 2012. "Techniques of functional and motility test: How to perform and interpret intestinal permeability." *Journal of Neurogastroenterology and Motility* 18(4):443–47.

Ravishankaran, P., and R. Karunanithi. 2011. "Clinical significance of preoperative serum interleukin-6 and C-reactive protein level in breast cancer patients." *World Journal of Surgical Oncology* 9:18.

Robbins, C. L., et al. 2009. "Influence of reproductive factors on mortality after epithelial ovarian cancer disgnosis." *Cancer Epidemiology, Biomarkers, and Prevention* 18(7):2035–41.

Salhab, M., S. Bismohun, and K. Mokbel. 2010. "Risk-reducing strategies for women carrying BRCA^1/$_2$ mutations with a focus on prophylactic surgery." *BMC Women's Health* (October 20):10–28.

Sandblom, G., et al. 2011. "Randomized prostate cancer screening trial: Twenty-year follow-up." *BMJ* 342:d1539.

Schalinske, K. L., and A. L. Smazal. 2012. "Homocysteine imbalance: A pathological metabolic marker." *Advances in Nutrition* 3(6):755–62.

Varker, K. A., C. E. Terrell, M. Welt, S. Suleiman, L. Thornton, B. L. Andersen, and W. E. Carson III. 2007. "Impaired natural killer cell lysis in breast cancer patients with high levels of psychological stress is associated with altered expression of killer immunoglobin-like receptors." *Journal of Surgical Research* 139(1):36–44.

Winchester, D. P. 2011. "Post-treatment surveillance of breast cancer patients in an organized, multidisciplinary setting." *Journal of Surgical Oncology* 103(4):358–61.

Wong, E. M., et al. 2011. "Constitutional methylation of the BRCA1 promoter is specifically associated with BRCA1 mutation-associated pathology in early-onset breast cancer." *Cancer Prevention Research* 4(1):23–33.

Zander, Rosamund, and Benjamin Zander. 2002. *The Art of Possibility: Transforming Professional and Personal Life.* New York: Penguin.

Acknowledgments

It is truly a gift and an honor to be able to write a book that people read, and more miraculous still, that inspires hope and health. I am grateful every day for the opportunity to offer this book to the world. Of course, central to this offering is the incredible talent, wisdom, and compassion of my coauthor, Karolyn Gazella. I am entirely grateful to have found such a wonderful person with whom to write. And, even better, we share a delightful friendship filled with laughter, teasing, encouragement, and a shared passion to create a healthier and happier world.

Writing is a very insular activity—one that demands many hours of uninterrupted time. It amazes me how gracefully and graciously my partner, Ann, has created a sequestered island in the middle of our busy lives for me to hide away on and write. She facilitates so much in our lives, and for this I am so very grateful. I also have to say that our four-legged companion Nora has lent her share to the effort. Her insistence to play ball, with complete disregard for my work, brings the joy of the moment into my days. Nora helps me stay balanced. Who is to say, at the end of the day, that a perfectly caught ball is not just as important as the completion of a paragraph?

Finally, I am spectacularly blessed with an incredible family. I have wise, kind, brave, and beautiful siblings—my sister Britt, my brother Alfie, and my sister Elena. I give thanks as well for my constant quest for understanding and realize that this comes honestly as I observe my ever-inquisitive Mom. And, finally, thank you, Dad, for being such a wonderful inspiration, father, and teacher—I hope your spirit continues to soar.

—L.A.

Each day I am grateful for the love that surfaces within and around me. I feel an awe-inspiring adoration for the beautiful nature that surrounds me, my lovely pup and two handsome horses, my friends, my family, and my work. To say that I am fortunate pales in comparison to how I really feel about this wonderful journey that I am on. More than a decade ago, I began working with a talented, inspired young doctor who has now become a close friend and business partner. Dr. Lise Alschuler is not only an exceptional writer and writing partner, but she is also a gifted speaker, teacher, and healer. I count Lise among my most cherished blessings.

In our lifetimes, we all should have at least one person that is always there no matter what; one person who loves us unconditionally; one person who helps us be the best we can be. That person in my life is my sister and best friend, Kathi Magee. I have immense respect, love, and gratitude for Kathi—she is my rock!

My work and my life have been influenced by many kind, talented, and wonderful people—far too many to list here, but you know who you are! You bring a smile to my face, you build me up when I am feeling down, you get the creative juices flowing, and I feel comfort and joy when I am in your presence. Thank you, friends; your love and support are so very much appreciated!

Finally, Lise and I appreciate the folks at Ten Speed Press and Random House for helping us make this second edition even better. We'd like to give a special thanks to Ten Speed editors Lisa Regul and Julie Bennett for their expertise and influence on this edition.

—K.G.

About the Authors

Dr. Lise N. Alschuler and Karolyn A. Gazella have been collaborating since 2002. Together they are the authors of *The Definitive Guide to Cancer*. They also host the popular Internet radio show *Five to Thrive Live!* featured on the Cancer Support Network at www.w4cs.com. For more information about them, visit www.FivetoThrivePlan.com.

Lise N. Alschuler, ND, FABNO, is a naturopathic doctor with board certification in naturopathic oncology. She graduated from Brown University with an undergraduate degree in medical anthropology and received her doctorate in naturopathic medicine from Bastyr University. Lise currently practices at Naturopathic Specialists, based in Scottsdale, Arizona. She is past president of the American Association of Naturopathic Physicians, is a founding board member of the Oncology Association of Naturopathic Physicians, and currently serves as a director on both the American Board of Naturopathic Oncology and the Naturopathic Post-Graduation Association. She is the vice president of quality and education at Emerson Ecologics, where she developed and manages the Emerson Quality Program—a rigorous quality assurance program for professional dietary supplement brands. She also works as an independent consultant in the area of practitioner and consumer health education.

Previously, Lise was the department head of naturopathic medicine at Midwestern Regional Medical Center–Cancer Treatment Centers of America, a Joint Commission on Accreditation of Healthcare Organizations–accredited regional hospital offering comprehensive integrative cancer care. Prior to that, she was the clinic medical director and botanical medicine chair at Bastyr University Natural Health Clinic. She is widely recognized as an expert in cancer treatment and prevention and is a sought-after speaker to physicians, patients, and the general public. While Lise was in clinical practice in Seattle, Washington, she was recognized as one of Seattle's "Top Doctors" by *Seattle Magazine*, she received the President's Award from the Oncology Association of Naturopathic Physicians, and she was named as one of the "Naturopathic Elders" by the Canadian College of Naturopathic Medicine. Lise is also a breast cancer survivor. For more information, visit www.drlise.net.

Karolyn A. Gazella is the publisher of the *Natural Medicine Journal*, an innovative peer-reviewed medical journal for holistic-minded health care practitioners (www.naturalmedicine journal.com). Karolyn has been writing and publishing wellness information since 1992. She is the author or coauthor of hundreds of articles and several books as well as the blog *The Healing Factor*, on PsychologyToday.com. In 2009, Karolyn was named one of the "Top 10 People in Integrative Health Care and Integrative Medicine" by the *Integrator Blog*. She is a volunteer for the Medicine Horse Program located in Boulder, Colorado, which is an innovative equine-assisted therapy program that helps high-risk youth. In 1995, Karolyn she was diagnosed with ovarian cancer. For more information, visit www.karolyngazella.com.

Index

outdoors, 53
requirements for, 41
starting, 52–53, 56–57
stretching and, 48–49
time of day for, 49–50
See also Fitness
MRIs (magnetic
resonance imaging),
155, 156–57
Muscle strengthening,
47–48
Myeloma, 114

N

National Cancer Institute,
44, 75
Natural killer (NK) cells,
12, 17, 34, 42,
59, 160
Neutrophils, 13
NF-kB (nuclear factor
kappa B), 14, 75,
112, 116
Nutritional
assessment, 167

O

Obesity, 66
Omega-3 fatty acids,
95–99
Optimism, 32–33
Organic foods, 70–72, 93
Ovarian cancer, 15,
32, 36, 60, 83–84,
152–53

P

Pancreatic cancer, 82,
113, 125
Pap tests, 153–54
Pedometers, 52
Pelvic exams. *See*
Gynecological
exams

Personality types, 145
Pessimism, 32–33
Pets, 56
Phthalates, 165
Pilates, 48, 49, 55
Playfulness, 142–43
Polyphenols, 75, 81,
105–18
Portion size, 66–67,
76–77
Prevention
antioxidants and,
121–22
approach to, 3
behavior change and,
6–8
curcumin and, 113–14
diet and, 61–62, 68, 73
green tea and, 106,
108–10
movement and, 44–45
omega-3 fatty acids
and, 96, 98
probiotics and, 103
resveratrol and, 117–18
vitamin D and, 125–27
See also Screening
Probiotics, 59, 100–105
Prostate cancer
curcumin and, 113
diet and, 60, 69, 75, 78,
82, 83
green tea and, 108
movement and, 44–45
omega-3 fatty acids
and, 98
screening for, 150–52
sleep and, 134
testosterone and, 15
vitamin D and,
125, 127
Protein, 77

PSA blood test, 150–52
Pterostilbene, 117

Q

Qi Gong, 55
Quercetin, 105

R

Radiation, 155
Rejuvenation
enhancing, 146
five critical action steps
for, 135–45
five key pathways and,
133–35
Five Rs of, 135–45
Relationships
loving, 36–37
reevaluating, 143–45
Relaxation, 133,
139–41, 146
Remediation, 143–45
Remen, Rachel Naomi,
34–35, 36
Replenishment, 141–43
Rest, 138–39. *See also*
Sleep
Resveratrol, 105, 115–18
Rhythm, 136–38
Risk assessment testing,
167–69
RNA, 172
Rosemary, 75

S

Sadness, 30
Screening
for breast cancer, 154,
156–57
for cervical and uterine
cancer, 153–54
for colon cancer,
149–50
goal of, 148